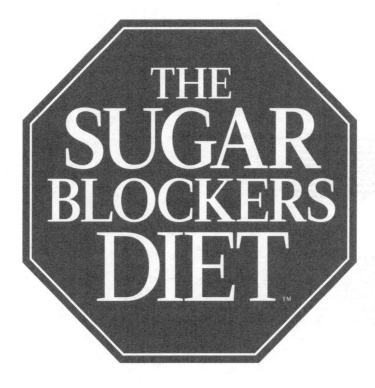

THE
SUGAR
BLOCKERS
DIET™

THE SUGAR BLOCKERS DIET™

ROB THOMPSON, MD,
WITH THE EDITORS OF **Prevention**

EAT GREAT, LOSE WEIGHT

A Doctor's 3-Step Plan to Lose Weight,
Lower Blood Sugar, and Beat Diabetes—
While Eating the Carbs You Love

RODALE.

Printed in the United States of America
Rodale Inc. makes every effort to use acid-free ♾, recycled paper ♻.

Exercise photos by Mitch Mandel/Rodale Images
Profile photos by Tom MacDonald/Rodale Images

Book design by Toby Fox

Library of Congress Cataloging-in-Publication Data

Thompson, Rob, 1945–
The sugar blockers diet : Eat great, lose weight. A doctor's 3-step plan to lose weight, lower blood sugar, and beat diabetes—while eating the carbs you love / Rob Thompson, with the editors of Prevention.
    p.   cm.
Includes bibliographical references and index.
ISBN 978-1-60961-253-5   direct hardcover
1. Reducing diets.   2. Non-insulin-dependent diabetes—Diet therapy.   3. Fiber in human nutrition.   4. Glycemic index.   I. Prevention Magazine Health Books.   II. Title.
    RM222.2.T4848   2011
613.2'5—dc23   2011037758

2   4   6   8   10   9   7   5   3   hardcover

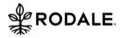

We inspire and enable people to improve their lives and the world around them
For more of our products, visit **prevention.com** or call 800-848-4735.

To Kathy

CONTENTS

INTRODUCTION

———•

A BOUT 12 YEARS AGO, on a trip out of town, I found myself getting up in the middle of the night with an unquenchable thirst and the need to urinate. I knew something was wrong and figured that diabetes was high on the list of possibilities. As a preventive cardiologist, I specialize in treating conditions that lead to heart disease, including diabetes. I have analyzers in my office for checking blood sugar, so I promised myself that I would check it when I got back to the office. When my medical assistant handed me the results, I was dumbfounded. My blood sugar wasn't just a little over the line—it was sky-high.

It's amazing how having a disease changes your perspective about it. As a physician, I spent my days making diagnoses, analyzing lab tests, and making decisions about medications. I gave overweight folks and those with diabetes advice about their diet and exercise habits but didn't spend much time thinking about it. That was *their* world. When I got diabetes, I suddenly entered that world. I had no problem figuring out what lab tests I needed or which medications to take, but every day I found myself grappling with a more primal aspect of life: what to eat. Having diabetes, I could never forget that the disease is a disturbance in the way the body handles food.

If you are overweight or have type 2 diabetes, the reasons are the same: Your pancreas has to make higher-than-normal amounts of the hormone insulin to keep your blood sugar down. Excessive insulin makes you fat, and producing all that insulin eventually wears out your insulin-making cells, which is when your blood sugar goes up.

Your body needs insulin to metabolize carbohydrates, foods that your digestive system turns to sugar. If you could stop eating carbs altogether, no doubt you'd lose weight, and if you have diabetes, your blood sugar would be a cinch to control. But cutting carbs is easier said than done. We like our fruits, vegetables, baked goods, and sweets. Isn't there an easier way than avoiding carbohydrates altogether?

Well, it turns out there is. If you're typical, you squander most of the insulin your body produces on surging blood sugar levels that occur immediately after meals. The fact is, you don't have to cut out all carbohydrates—only the ones that cause these "sugar shocks." Scientists now rate carbohydrates according to their glycemic load—how high they shoot up your blood sugar right after you eat them. The good news is that only a handful of foods have glycemic loads high enough to cause sugar shocks. The bad news is, they're some of our favorite foods. We're used to eating them at virtually every meal.

That's where sugar blockers come in. There are ways that you can blunt the blood sugar–raising effects of carbohydrates. For example, many of our favorite foods contain substances that interfere with the breakdown of carbohydrates to sugar in your digestive tract and slow its absorption into your bloodstream. Not only do these natural sugar-blocking substances inhibit the absorption of sugar in the foods that contain them, but they also block the absorption of sugar in other foods that you eat with them. You don't have to avoid carbs completely if you combine them with foods that contain these sugar blockers.

Adding sugar-blocking foods to your diet isn't the only way to lessen after-meal sugar spikes. The order in which you eat food, your activities before and after you eat, how much fluid you drink with your meal, the time of day, and even the amount of sleep you get—all affect how high your blood sugar goes after you eat a carbohydrate. In addition, the pharmaceutical industry has recently developed revolutionary new sugar-blocking medications that slow the entry of sugar into your bloodstream, reduce your body's needs for insulin, and reliably produce significant and lasting weight loss.

None of these sugar blockers will completely prevent the rise in blood sugar and insulin demands that occurs after you eat a starchy carbohydrate. However, they *can* decrease it significantly, and researchers have discovered that it doesn't take much sugar blocking to provide benefits. Reducing the size of after-meal blood sugar spikes by just 30 percent reduces insulin demands, promotes weight loss, makes diabetes easier to control, and can actually reverse prediabetes. Most remarkable, recent studies have shown significant reductions in the incidence of heart disease among both followers of low–glycemic load diets and people who take pharmaceutical sugar blockers.

I have been using the methods described in this book for years. My diabetes has remained in excellent control, I lost the 25 extra pounds I was carrying around, and truly, I eat better now than ever. I also recommend this approach to my patients. Recently the editors of *Prevention* and I invited a select group of men and women interested in losing weight to try it, and we closely tracked their progress. Our panel of testers didn't count calories, limit fat or sugar, or try to reduce the amount of food that they ate. Actually, they were amazed at how easy it was to fit sugar blockers into their life. Cindy Swan, 59, reported, "I never felt like I was starving or missing out." Nancy Mikkelsen, 53, concurred: "It wasn't this enormous, radical change that had to happen. It was small things that obviously made a difference. . . . It just makes sense."

And their results were impressive. Of the 16 people who tried the plan, all but one lost weight. Valerie Hayes, 53, lost 18$\frac{1}{2}$ pounds and 9$\frac{1}{4}$ inches total in her waist, chest, hip, thighs, and arms in 6 weeks on the plan, and

Linda Frey, 52, lost 17$^1/_2$ pounds and 13$^3/_4$ inches. It wasn't just their weight that improved. Most of the panelists also saw their blood sugar levels, blood pressure, and triglyceride levels come down—including one by an incredible 500 points. Many reported that their moods and energy levels improved.

It was gratifying to see these panelists reduce their risk for type 2 diabetes and heart disease, drop pounds, and have energy to spare, all while enjoying most of their favorite foods. Throughout the book you'll read some of their inspiring stories, along with their practical tips on how to make sugar blocking second nature, as told to the editors of *Prevention* magazine.

My hope in writing this book is to take you beyond the grind of just trying to avoid carbohydrates and introduce you to ways that you can change how they behave in your body. I'll show you how to put different sugar-blocking foods and strategies to work to lower your blood sugar and correct the metabolic disturbances that make you gain weight. Admittedly, it's a rough science, and we're only beginning to understand it. However, if you're trying to lose weight or control diabetes, I think you'll find that learning how sugar blocking works will not only help you accomplish your weight loss and blood sugar goals but also make your diet tastier and your life easier.

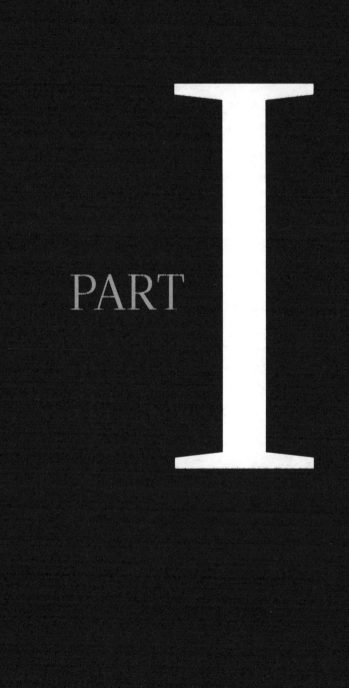

PART I

WHY SUGAR BLOCK?

ALBERT EINSTEIN is credited with saying that the definition of insanity is when you keep trying the same thing over and over again while expecting different results. Despite steadily rising obesity and diabetes rates, nutritionists keep passing out the same advice—cut fat, cut cholesterol, don't eat so much—expecting that somehow the results will be different. Of course, when the advice doesn't work, you can always blame the recipient's lack of willpower. However, twice as many of us are overweight today as were overweight 30 years ago. Did we all suddenly lose our willpower?

Well, the proof is in: The advice we've been getting for the past 40 years doesn't work.

In Part I we clear our minds of old notions, take a look at what medical science has learned in the past decades, and engage in some fresh thinking about obesity and its henchman, type 2 diabetes. The first chapter traces our problems back to their beginning and pinpoints what changed to bring them on. Chapter 2 shows you how a hormone you can't live without can work against you. Chapter 3 identifies the cause of the excessive demands for insulin that make you gain weight and wear out your insulin-making cells. In Chapter 4, you'll see how slowing the absorption of starch into your bloodstream is the key to alleviating excessive insulin demands, losing weight, and preventing or treating diabetes.

1

CARBOHYDRATES
AND THE
DISEASES OF
CIVILIZATION

DON'T EAT THIS, don't eat that. You might not even listen anymore. Sure, if you swore off all carbohydrates—sugar, flour products, potatoes, rice, fruit and fruit juice, vegetables, and soft drinks—you'd lose weight. And if you have diabetes, it would be a lot easier to control. But you've also been told that you should avoid fat and cholesterol: eggs, butter, cheese, red meat, and so on, not to mention salt and trans fats. It's enough to drive you crazy. If you followed all the dietary advice you hear these days, you'd hardly have anything left to eat—fish and lettuce, maybe.

Take a deep breath. Here's how a preventive cardiologist—who specializes in treating diabetes, obesity, and heart disease and has followed diet research for 30 years—sees it: It doesn't matter if you're a strict vegetarian, a voracious carnivore, or an incurable chocoholic. The important thing is that you *block sugar*.

Block sugar? You've probably never heard of it, but that's what it boils down to. The single most consistent finding that has emerged from diet research in the past 30 years is this: The best way to lose weight, prevent or treat diabetes, improve the balance between good and bad blood cholesterol, and prevent heart disease is to do things to inhibit the breakdown of carbohydrates to sugar in your digestive tract and slow its entry into your bloodstream.

Let me explain.

● LOW-CARB LIVING, STONE AGE–STYLE

The foods we eat contain three major nutrients: fats, proteins, and carbohydrates. Each has its own building blocks: Fats are made of fatty acids, proteins consist of amino acids, and carbohydrates are made of a type of sugar called glucose. Fat and protein come primarily from animal products such as eggs, meat, and dairy products, and from oily foods like nuts and olives. You get carbohydrates from plant products, including fruits, vegetables, flour, potatoes, rice, and sugar. Your digestive tract has to break down each kind of food to its basic building blocks—either fatty acids, amino acids, or glucose—before it can be absorbed into your bloodstream.

If you're typical of most modern humans, you get most of your calories from carbohydrates—foods that your digestive system breaks down into glucose. However, we didn't always eat this way. Prehistoric humans mainly ate other creatures—large ones, small ones, fish, and even bugs. The plants they consumed—grasses, roots, and wild fruit in various stages of ripeness—contained plenty of vitamins but yielded little in the way of calories. That's because natural vegetation is full of indigestible fiber and other substances that interfere with the breakdown of carbohydrates to glucose and prevent their absorption into the bloodstream. The digestive tracts of our ancient ancestors had to work hard to digest the plants they ate. Whatever glucose they absorbed trickled into their bloodstream over several hours. Most of the vegetation they consumed passed through their intestines undigested.

STARCH: NATURE'S Rocket Fuel

HOW DO seeds get energy to sprout if they're underground and don't have leaves to soak up sunlight? Nature solves this problem by loading up seeds with a powerful fuel: starch. Starch is nothing but sugar molecules linked end to end by flimsy bonds, which plant and animal enzymes have no trouble breaking. Starch looks like a white powder, but it's actually chains of glucose molecules stacked together like cordwood to form tiny crystals loaded with caloric energy. No food we commonly eat, *including fat,* has as many calories packed into as small a space as starch.

The funny thing is, you can't taste it. Starch doesn't turn to sugar until it reaches your gut, where it is quickly broken down and absorbed into your bloodstream.

About 10,000 years ago, the human diet changed dramatically. In an area known as the Fertile Crescent in what are now parts of Iraq and Syria, wild wheat and barley grew in abundance. The seeds of those grasses contain unusually large amounts of starch, a powdery substance that consists of glucose molecules linked together in long chains. Enzymes in the seeds can break the bonds that hold the starch molecules together and use the glucose for the energy needed to sprout. The high starch content of these seeds gave them a jump start so they could mature quickly during the short rainy season typical of this region.

Although Mother Nature intended starch to be used as an energy source for plants, not animals, the bonds that hold its glucose molecules together are weak enough that the digestive enzymes of animals can break them, too. To keep predators from eating the starch in these seeds, they were encased in rock-hard husks. You can't just strip wheat seeds from the stalk and eat them; you'd break your teeth. Somehow you have to extract the starch from the husk.

About 10,000 years ago, some of our more resourceful ancestors learned to grind wheat and barley seeds between rocks and let the wind blow away the chaff. This crude bit of technology gave humans access to a huge, previously untapped source of easily digestible calories. Best of all, unlike most of the other foods they ate, grains could be stored between growing seasons and provide food year-round.

As time passed, a similar event occurred in the Far East, where humans learned to extract rice and millet kernels from their husks. Later, Native Americans introduced European settlers to corn—another edible grain—and to the potato, which is also packed with starch.

It didn't take long for our ancestors to figure out that starches, such as wheat, rice, corn, and potatoes, could feed more people more dependably

THE ECONOMICS OF STARCH:
WHY WE EAT So Much of It

THE REASON we consume so much starch is that it's cheap. Starch crops such as wheat, potatoes, rice, and corn can provide more calories with less investment of land, labor, and capital than any other kind of food. Not only is starchy food cheap for you, but it's also cheap for restaurants and food manufacturers who prepare food for you. Whenever you pay for food prepared by others, they profit by using cheap ingredients. That's why restaurants are happy to serve you free bread before your meal and a large baked potato with it.

The best way to make money selling food is to use cheap ingredients and charge a high price. Starch is cheap enough. The trick is to sell it at a high price. As it happens, food manufacturers can often obtain patents on their processing tech-niques, which bar other companies from making the same product. That allows processed-food manufacturers to charge whatever price they want to without fear of being undercut by competitors. Then all they have to do is convince people to buy their products. The large markups of price over produc-tion costs that are typical of patented processed foods allow for big advertising budgets. That's why you see lots of TV commercials for break-fast cereals, potato chips, and crackers but not for fresh fruit, vegetables, meat, and dairy prod-ucts. You can't obtain patents for fresh produce, so there's nothing to keep the competition from driving prices down, and profit margins are too small to allow for large advertis-ing budgets.

and easily than any other kind of food. The agricultural way of life soon supplanted the hunter-gatherer existence. Instead of relying on fat and protein for calories as their preagricultural ancestors had for millions of years, humans started eating more carbohydrates—a lot more. We modern humans now consume *hundreds of times* more digestible glucose molecules than our ancient ancestors did, and starches provide most of the calories for most of the people in the world.

LEARN THE LINGO:
Carbohydrate Terminology

PLANTS MANUFACTURE the sugar glucose literally out of thin air by combining carbon dioxide in the air with water from the soil, using energy from sunlight. Glucose is the building block of all plant life.

Most of the glucose molecules in plants and trees are connected by unbreakable *beta* bonds that form the structural material for leaves, branches, roots, etc. However, the glucose molecules in starch are linked together by weak *alpha* bonds, which are easy for the enzymes of plants and animals to break, providing a ready source of energy.

Both plants and animals change some glucose to fructose, a sugar that is almost identical to glucose except for a slight rearrangement of atoms. Plants also produce the sugar sucrose, a double molecule comprising one glucose molecule linked to one fructose molecule. Cane sugar, the type of sugar we use to sweeten our coffee and tea, is pure sucrose. The digestive tract breaks down sucrose into glucose and fructose before it is absorbed into the bloodstream.

When laypeople use the word *sugar,* they are usually referring to cane sugar—that is, sucrose. However, when doctors use the term *blood sugar,* they usually mean glucose. This creates some confusion: It leads people to think that diabetes comes from eating too much sugar, the kind you put in coffee or tea. Some people even call diabetes "sugar diabetes." In fact, most of the sugar in people's blood does not come from sucrose, it comes from the breakdown of starch. According to the Nurses' Health Study, a survey of the diets of more than 121,700 women, Americans get several times more glucose from starch than from sucrose. A more appropriate term would be *starch diabetes.*

● THE DISEASES OF CIVILIZATION

With the advent of agriculture, human beings no longer had to be constantly on the move searching for food. Once they learned to plant crops, they settled down and began to form communities and, eventually, the beginnings of civilization as we know it today. The cultivation of starches fostered agricultural-based societies that would come to dominate the world.

But there was a price to pay for our progress. The digestive systems of all animals are designed to handle diets specific to each species. For example, the digestive systems of herbivores, such as deer, are designed for eating grasses and leaves. Similarly, the digestive systems of carnivores, such as cats, are designed for eating meat; carnivores can't live on vegetation. Indeed, the cure for diabetes and obesity in pet cats is to stop feeding them grain-based commercial cat food and let them return to eating pure meat.

It's not surprising that the dramatic shift from the hunter-gatherer diet of meat and crude vegetation to a diet based largely on starches had profound effects on human health. In fact, when humans gave up the hunter-gatherer lifestyle and began consuming more carbohydrates, they became shorter in stature, less muscular, and prone to what scientists call diseases of civilization, including obesity, diabetes, and heart disease.

What was it about the change in diet brought on by the advent of agriculture that caused these problems? It's not that human beings had never eaten carbohydrates before. Some of our *really* ancient ancestors—apes and monkeys—lived on vegetation. The difference is that the plant parts we consume have become increasingly *refined*—that is, stripped of their natural barriers to digestion. The rates of obesity, diabetes, and heart disease correlate directly with the lack of inhibitors to carbohydrate absorption in the diet. Today Americans who consume below-average amounts of natural sugar-blocking substances have significantly higher rates of obesity, diabetes, and heart disease than do those who consume larger amounts. What is it about stripping plants of their natural barriers to digestion that makes us prone to those problems?

It has to do with the hormone insulin.

2

INSULIN: THE CALORIE-STORING HORMONE

REACH DOWN and grab a handful of your belly fat. There you go. Now ask yourself, with all that fat, *why in the world would you ever be hungry?* Why doesn't your body just use the calories you have stored up in your fat for energy?

The reason: insulin.

No one needs to be convinced that we Americans have a weight problem; just look around you. Two-thirds of us are fat enough to increase our risk of diabetes and heart disease. A third of us are obese—30 pounds overweight or more.

We didn't used to be so chunky. Look at photographs from the 1960s. The incidence of obesity in the United States then was less than half of what it is now, and it had been the same for years. Then, around 1970, the obesity rate suddenly started rising. Since then, the number of overweight and obese Americans doubled. What happened?

● DIABESITY

Until recently, obesity got short shrift when it came to scientific research. Doctors worried more about *under*nutrition. However, one condition that doctors have always taken seriously is diabetes. In fact, along with the skyrocketing obesity rate since 1970 has come an epidemic of diabetes in adults. As scientists learned more about the causes of diabetes, it has become apparent that adult-onset diabetes and obesity are just different manifestations of the same disease process. Some doctors call it *diabesity*. Indeed, if you come to understand what brings on adult-onset diabetes, you'll also see why so many people these days are overweight.

Diabetes occurs when your body loses its ability to keep your blood sugar levels from rising too high. There are two distinct kinds: type 1, or juvenile-onset, diabetes; and type 2, or adult-onset, diabetes. Type 1 tends to strike children and young adults. It's caused by damage to the body's insulin-making cells—the beta cells of the pancreas—brought on by an immune-system reaction to an infection. Insulin transports sugar out of your blood and into your cells, where it is either stored as fat or used for energy. If you don't make enough insulin, sugar backs up in your bloodstream. For people with type 1 diabetes, high blood sugar is purely the result of a lack of insulin. Otherwise, the body chemistry functions normally.

In the past, children and young people with type 1 diabetes often died for lack of insulin. Insulin shots, which became available in the 1920s, were a godsend for these patients. Although getting medicinal insulin into the system the same way that normal beta cells do it can be challenging, correcting the deficiency makes the body chemistry function normally again and prevents most of the complications of juvenile diabetes. Insulin allows people with type 1 diabetes to live normal lives.

The development of insulin as medication is one of the seminal achievements of modern medicine. It has saved millions of lives. Understandably, it has had a profound effect on the public's and the medical profession's perceptions of diabetes. Indeed, the word *diabetes* has become synonymous with lack of insulin. However, you will see that this is misleading. The fact is that most people with type 2 diabetes actually make *too much* insulin.

In contrast with patients who have type 1 diabetes, those with type 2 diabetes often don't need insulin to control their blood sugar. In the past, doctors thought that adult-onset diabetes was just a milder form of the kind that kids get—also caused by a lack of insulin—but not as severe a deficiency. Then, in the 1980s, scientists made a remarkable discovery: The beta cells of patients with type 2 diabetes produce plenty of insulin. The problem is that their bodies lose sensitivity to it, a condition called insulin resistance. Consequently, the beta cells have to make greater-than-normal amounts of insulin to compensate for the body's loss of sensitivity to it.

● WHEN THE BODY STOPS RESPONDING TO INSULIN

Remember, your body doesn't need much insulin to handle fat and protein. You need it mainly to metabolize carbohydrates—foods your digestive tract turns to sugar. If you have insulin resistance, your body has to produce unnaturally large amounts of insulin to handle the carbohydrates in your diet. Insulin keeps trying to transport glucose out of your blood and into your cells, but your cells no longer respond properly to it.

Insulin resistance goes on for years before diabetes occurs. At first your beta cells are able to produce enough extra insulin to compensate for your body's lack of sensitivity to it. However, as the years pass, the beta cells wear out from overuse, and their ability to sustain such high levels of insulin production gradually dwindles. When they can no longer keep up with your body's excessive demands for insulin, your blood sugar rises, which is when doctors make the diagnosis of diabetes.

AMYLIN: INSULIN'S Evil Fraternal Twin

EVERY TIME your beta cells make a molecule of insulin, they also produce a molecule of a by-product called amylin. Amylin actually helps insulin lower blood sugar. However, excessive amounts of amylin can accumulate in your beta cells and form an insoluble sludge called amyloid.

Buildup of amyloid irreversibly damages beta cells.

Some scientists call amylin "insulin's evil fraternal twin." Amyloid buildup in beta cells caused by years of excessive insulin and amylin production is one reason type 2 diabetes, although preventable, is difficult to reverse once you get it.

You see, then, that a crucial difference between type 1 and type 2 diabetes is that, while people with type 1 diabetes have trouble handling carbohydrates, carbs don't actually *cause* the disease—it's triggered by an immune reaction to an infection. On the other hand, the unnaturally large amounts of refined carbohydrates typical of the modern diet, coupled with insulin resistance, wear out your beta cells and bring on type 2 diabetes.

Approximately 40 percent of Americans these days eventually develop insulin resistance. However, only a minority of people with insulin resistance go on to develop diabetes. Genetic factors, as well as influences that scientists are still unraveling, cause some people's beta cells to wear out faster than those of others.

Now, back to the question of why you get hungry even though you have plenty of calories stored up as fat. Although most people with insulin resistance continue making enough insulin to keep them from developing diabetes, they often develop other problems caused by excessive insulin secretion, the most frustrating of which is weight gain.

Here's how insulin resistance makes you fat: As you become insulin resistant, some parts of your body lose sensitivity to insulin, while others remain sensitive. This creates an imbalance. The unnaturally large amounts of insulin that your body has to make to overcome insulin resistance in the parts of your system that lose sensitivity *end up overloading the parts that are still sensitive.*

One part of your body that stays particularly sensitive to insulin is your fat cells. Fat is where the body stores calories, and insulin is the body's main calorie-storing hormone. Insulin pushes calories—whether from fat, protein, or carbohydrates—into your fat cells.

Normally, between meals fat flows out of your fat cells and into your bloodstream to provide energy and keep you from getting hungry. However, excessive amounts of insulin in your bloodstream virtually lock fat into your fat cells so that your body can't use it for energy. This creates a frustrating paradox: Even though you have plenty of calories stored up as fat, you seem to be hungry all of the time. Scientists call this internal starvation. Your fat starts acting like a giant tumor, robbing you of nutrition as it grows.

And fat, indeed, *does* tend to grow. Obesity actually makes insulin resistance worse, creating a vicious cycle: More insulin resistance promotes weight gain, which causes more insulin resistance and more weight gain.

● WHAT CAUSES INSULIN RESISTANCE?

Loss of sensitivity to insulin is not a problem with some internal organs, like your kidneys, liver, or spleen. *It's a muscle problem.* Your muscles are the major users of glucose and the target of most of the insulin that your body produces. The reason you lose sensitivity to insulin is that your muscles lose sensitivity to it, and the reason your muscles lose sensitivity to it is simply that *you don't use them enough.*

A hundred years ago, Americans consumed more calories and, in fact, more carbs than we do today, but obesity and type 2 diabetes were rare. Why? *Because people were more physically active.* It's hard to imagine how sedentary we are compared with previous generations. As recently as 1900, the majority of Americans lived and worked on farms. Even people who lived in cities were more active because motorized transportation hadn't taken over the job of moving them from one place to another. Folks thought nothing of walking several miles a day to go to school or work. Now we ride to work in cars and buses, sit at desks all day, ride home in cars and buses, and spend our evenings in front of our television sets and computers. Never in history have humans been as sedentary as we are today. Indeed, there would be no diabesity epidemic if we were as physically active as our 19th-century ancestors. Insulin resistance brought on by lack of physical activity set the stage for America's epidemic of obesity and type 2 diabetes.

The cure for insulin resistance—the only real cure—is exercise. Muscular activity turns the vicious cycle of insulin resistance into a virtuous cycle. It restores insulin sensitivity, which lowers insulin levels, which promotes weight loss, which further increases insulin sensitivity.

Many of us try to exercise, and any exercise is better than none. However, for relieving insulin resistance, some kinds of physical activity are more effective than others. It turns out that our efforts to exercise are often off the mark when it comes to losing weight and preventing diabetes. Here's the good news: You don't have to engage in grueling workouts to restore your muscles' sensitivity to insulin. Chapter 11, Exercise: Getting the Most Benefit with the Least Effort, will show you how to craft an exercise program directed not necessarily at building big muscles or winning foot races but at sensitizing your muscles to insulin, losing weight, and preventing or treating diabetes—in as little as 20 minutes a day.

Remember, though, that insulin resistance is only half the problem; it alone won't make you fat and diabetic. Only when insulin resistance is combined with a diet high in refined carbohydrates does it become a problem. That's why the incidences of obesity and diabetes have risen so sharply in the past four decades. Contrary to popular perception, Americans are eating less fat and cholesterol than we did 30 years ago, but we're eating more starch than ever. According to USDA statistics, flour consumption per person is up 48 percent, rice consumption is up 186 percent, and consumption of frozen potato products (mainly french fries) is up 131 percent since 1970. We have become a nation of starch eaters.

● ARE YOU INSULIN RESISTANT?

Directly measuring the body's sensitivity to insulin requires sophisticated testing techniques available only in dedicated research laboratories. However, doctors have learned to recognize insulin resistance with a few remarkably simple tests. If you have any three of the following signs, the odds are about five to one that you have insulin resistance.

▶ An abdominal girth measured at your navel of 38 inches or more if you are male, 34 inches if you are female. (Note: Your pants size is not an accurate measure of your abdominal girth. You need to wrap a tape measure around your belly at the level of your navel.)

▶ A blood triglyceride level of 150 or greater

▶ An HDL ("good cholesterol") level of less than 40 if you are male, less than 50 if you are female

Potbellies

ONE OF THE BEST ways to detect insulin resistance is to measure your abdominal girth. Insulin tends to pack calories into your belly fat as opposed to the fat on your buttocks, arms, or legs. People with insulin resistance tend to have what's commonly known as a potbelly. Excess abdominal fat has been linked to type 2 diabetes and heart disease.

Fat cells do more than store calories. They produce several hormones, some of which, in excess, can reduce insulin sensitivity and inflame blood vessels. Some scientists believe that because blood coming from the abdomen drains directly into the liver, excess abdominal fat is especially likely to worsen insulin resistance and may even cause it.

Using a scanning technique called positron-emission tomography (PET), scientists can see where fat is stored after we eat different foods. Indeed, while calories from fat and protein are stored all over the body, carbs go right to the belly.

- Blood pressure of 130/85 or higher

- Fasting blood sugar greater than 105

If you have three or more of those signs, chances are your body needs higher-than-normal amounts of insulin to handle the carbohydrates in your diet. If you wonder why you seem to be hungry all the time even though you have plenty of calories stored up as fat, there's your answer. Excessive insulin is locking calories in your fat stores so that the rest of your body can't use them to stave off hunger. You're in a state of internal starvation.

● THE HEART CONNECTION

Although virtually everybody with type 2 diabetes first develops insulin resistance, not everybody with insulin resistance develops diabetes. Among those who do not, beta cells seem to be able to handle the increased workload imposed by loss of sensitivity to insulin and excessive carbohydrate consumption. However, insulin resistance causes several metabolic problems that raise the risk of heart disease and stroke, *even if it doesn't bring on diabetes.*

High blood triglyceride. Loss of sensitivity to insulin, combined with amounts of refined carbohydrates typical of the modern diet, raises the levels of a type of fat in your blood called triglyceride. Triglyceride is your body's way of dealing with excessive carbohydrates. To keep glucose from building up in the blood, your liver changes it to fat and sends it through the bloodstream to your fat stores in the form of triglyceride.

Low levels of good cholesterol. A little triglyceride in your blood is normal, but too much of it causes problems. Although triglyceride doesn't damage arteries directly, it lowers blood levels of HDL, or "good cholesterol," a type of particle that actually removes cholesterol from your arteries. Low levels of good cholesterol raise the risk of heart attack and strokes, just as high levels of bad cholesterol do.

Increased numbers of bad-cholesterol particles. Cholesterol travels through your blood in packets called LDL, or "bad cholesterol." These are the particles that infiltrate your blood vessels and cause damage. Insulin resistance causes your liver to make more bad-cholesterol particles, but often these packets are smaller than normal. This creates some confusion when measuring cholesterol levels in the blood. Because the packets are smaller, each one carries less cholesterol, so even though there are more particles, often there is little change in the total amount of cholesterol in the blood. As it turns out, the risk of heart attack and stroke correlates better with the number of cholesterol packets in the blood than with the actual level of cholesterol. In other words, even though your cholesterol level is normal, you might have too many cholesterol particles in your blood.

High blood pressure. Insulin resistance, combined with large amounts of refined carbohydrates, raises blood pressure. It does this directly through its effects on your kidneys and blood vessels, and indirectly by causing weight gain. Reducing insulin excess by restoring insulin sensitivity with exercise and limiting refined carbohydrates lowers blood pressure.

Free-radical damage. Once doctors learned to recognize insulin resistance, they soon noticed its association with diabetes, cholesterol problems, and high blood pressure. Those things are easy to measure. However, researchers later discovered other harmful effects of insulin resistance that weren't so easy to recognize. As your body metabolizes glucose, it produces toxic by-products called free radicals, which in high concentrations damage arteries. Normally your body neutralizes these substances before they cause trouble, but sudden spikes in blood sugar and insulin levels cause excessive free-radical production, overwhelming the mechanisms that neutralize them and further contributing to artery damage.

HIGH BLOOD-TRIGLYCERIDE LEVELS: A WINDOW TO YOUR Carbohydrate Metabolism

THE TWO major fats in your blood are triglyceride and cholesterol. Whereas cholesterol can seep into your arteries and cause trouble, triglyceride is not directly damaging to blood vessels. However, in high concentrations, triglyceride "washes away" good cholesterol (HDL) and reduces its levels. Low levels of good cholesterol can be as harmful to arteries as increased levels of bad cholesterol.

Most doctors regard triglyceride levels of less than 150 as normal, concentrations between 150 and 200 as mildly elevated, and levels greater than 200 as high.

Triglyceride elevations are one of the most common laboratory abnormalities that doctors see, affecting approximately a third of Americans. Although mild increases are largely harmless, they are a sensitive indicator that something is amiss. Some diseases and medications can raise triglyceride levels, but the usual cause is a combination of insulin resistance and excessive consumption of refined carbohydrates.

If you do what you need to do to maintain normal triglyceride levels, chances are the other problems associated with insulin resistance—weight gain, low levels of good cholesterol, high blood pressure, and high blood sugar—will improve.

Enhanced clotting. Insulin resistance also raises levels of substances in the blood that increase its tendency to clot, which adds to the risk of heart attack and stroke.

● INSULIN: TOO MUCH OF A GOOD THING

In the past, it seemed to doctors that most type 2 diabetics could keep their blood sugar levels under control just by watching their diet and taking pills. Their mildly elevated blood sugar levels, although persistent, didn't seem to bother them much. Doctors seldom prescribed insulin shots for type 2 diabetics. They figured it wasn't worth the trouble.

In the 1990s, that laid-back approach to treating type 2 diabetes changed. Research showed that while folks with type 2 diabetes rarely died directly from high blood sugar, as patients with type 1 diabetes did, after several years they often developed the same kind of eye, nerve, and kidney damage. Most alarming, they suffered from heart attacks and strokes at rates several times higher than the general population. Most disappointing, the pills and diets that doctors were prescribing did little to prevent those complications.

Consequently, doctors started taking type 2 diabetes more seriously. They began prescribing stronger pills, and even insulin, to lower blood sugar levels further. A large, meticulously conducted research study, the United Kingdom Prospective Diabetes Study, found that better control of blood sugar indeed helps patients with type 2 diabetes avoid eye, nerve, and kidney damage. However, although research showed that lowering blood sugar with stronger medications prevented heart disease in those with type 1 diabetes, it didn't seem to do the same for patients with type 2 diabetes. Why would stronger medication prevent heart problems in those with type 1 diabetes but not type 2?

How well insulin works to prevent artery damage depends on what kinds of arteries you're trying to protect. You have two types of arteries in your body: big, thick ones, which carry blood to the various parts of your body; and tiny, delicate ones, which allow nutrients to sift out into your tissues. Diabetes damages eyes, nerves, and kidneys through its effects on those tiny, delicate arteries. It causes heart attacks and strokes by damaging the big, thick ones. As it turns out, lowering blood sugar by any means, including taking large doses of insulin, prevents damage to those small, delicate arteries, but it doesn't work nearly as well in protecting the big ones.

Many diabetes experts thought that if patients with type 2 diabetes just took more insulin and lowered their blood sugar to normal levels, the results would be better—that heart attacks and strokes would be prevented. To test this assumption, researchers conducted a large study called the Action to Control Cardiovascular Risk in Diabetes trial, nicknamed the ACCORD trial, which enrolled more than 10,000 people with type 2 diabetes. Researchers gave half of the patients standard treatment with pills and insulin, and the other half larger doses of insulin to bring down blood sugar levels to as close to normal as possible.

The results were disturbing. Trying to lower blood sugar to normal by giving more insulin not only caused more weight gain and episodes of dangerously low blood sugar but also resulted in *more* heart attacks. The study had to be stopped earlier than planned because of the danger that high doses of insulin posed to the participants.

● INSULIN: FRIEND AND ENEMY

Why would taking more insulin actually *increase* the risk of heart attack? The problem is that type 2 diabetes is an entirely different disease from type 1. For adults with type 2 diabetes, a lack of insulin isn't the problem; as you know by now, they usually make more than normal amounts of insulin. Taking more insulin lowers blood sugar but often just adds to an existing excess of insulin and does nothing to correct what brings on type 2 diabetes in the first place—loss of sensitivity to insulin and the unnaturally large amounts of rapidly digestible carbohydrates typical of the modern diet. Although insulin lowers blood sugar, which is a good thing, excessive amounts of insulin and glucose can cause cholesterol imbalance, raise blood pressure, generate free radicals, and trigger overactive blood clotting, all conditions that damage large blood vessels.

Another problem is that treating high blood sugar with ever-larger doses of insulin causes weight gain, which invariably makes diabetes more difficult to control. The patients in the ACCORD trial who took the larger doses of insulin gained more weight than the ones who took smaller amounts. Ironically, then, by trying to control blood sugar by taking more insulin, you can end up gaining weight and making it harder to control.

Any doctor will tell you that the four most powerful risk factors for heart attacks and strokes are the following:

▶ Imbalance between good and bad cholesterol

▶ High blood pressure

▶ High blood sugar

▶ Cigarette smoking

Rarely does anyone have a heart attack without at least one of those risk factors present. Considering that high insulin levels in the blood, whether from medication or from being secreted naturally, are associated with three of the four biggest risk factors for heart attack, it's not surprising that the large doses of insulin used in ACCORD actually raised the risk.

That's not to say that insulin isn't useful for treating type 2 diabetes. In fact, taking insulin is one of the best things you can do if you have type 2 diabetes. In addition to lowering blood sugar, it relieves overworked beta cells of some of their burden and helps keep them from wearing out. Make no mistake: Insulin per se isn't the problem; it's the *unnaturally large amounts of insulin* needed to overcome insulin resistance and excessive dietary carbohydrates that cause trouble.

One thing that's true of hormones in general is that they need to be carefully regulated. Too little of them causes trouble; too much causes trouble. The ACCORD trial reminded doctors that insulin—whether the body's own or insulin taken as medication—is no different from any other hormone. It can work for you or against you. It always lowers blood sugar, which is a good thing, but too much of it causes trouble. If you want to lose weight or control type 2 diabetes, the most important thing to do is to try to eliminate the two problems that raise your body's demand for insulin in the first place: insulin resistance and too much glucose rushing into your bloodstream too fast—what you might call "sugar shocks."

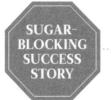
Age: 58

Height: 5' 6"

Pounds lost: 18½

Inches lost: 9¼

Major accomplishment:
Improved all three major health markers (blood sugar, blood pressure, and cholesterol), including shedding 33 points of LDL cholesterol!

Favorite sugar blockers:
Chia seeds

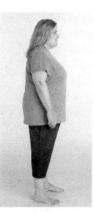

before

VALERIE HAYES
Saying Good-Bye to Starch

AS HER 58TH BIRTHDAY approached, Valerie Hayes was pushing 250 pounds—and becoming aware of some key concerns. For one, diabetes runs in her family. Second, her weight alone put her at risk for the disease. And third, diabetes can sneak up on anyone. In fact, the sleuth factor of this near epidemic is what helped motivate Valerie to try the Sugar Blockers Diet. She wanted to learn more about diabetes because she knew it was "quite sneaky."

Valerie took a step in the right direction. Knowledge is power, and with the program she found the power she needed to get her health back on track and reach her weight loss goal of more than 15 pounds. "It created a consistency in my day," she said of the program. "I had never been used to eating three meals. I sleep more regularly. Eating three meals and planning out my day was a good thing—it made me more efficient, following some regularity. [Before the program] I would eat anytime, [in the] middle of the night."

The routine helped not only her diet but also her workout routine. Prior to the Sugar Blockers Diet, Valerie said, she did exercise, just not consistently. And as the years went by, it started to seem as if her days of bike riding, skiing, and kayaking were becoming more like annual or special events rather than regular exercise.

Fortunately, the completion of the Delaware & Lehigh National Heritage Trail (conveniently located in front of Valerie's home) coincided with her decision to find out more about diabetes and stop the approach of the disease. She signed up for trail patrol and ordered Nordic walking poles. "I loved them," she said. "I think they [are what] helped burn off the calories. A little kid called me an old lady, but I don't care." Before she knew it, Valerie was using her walking poles almost every day—and today could probably walk circles around any chuckling little children.

Now the diet-and-exercise routine has become how she lives her day, and 4 months after the program's end, Valerie's weight loss was approaching 40 pounds—more than twice as much as her original goal. Add in stabilized blood sugars and dramatic drops in cholesterol and triglyceride levels, and Valerie is well on her way to a healthier, diabetes-free life.

And she never thought of sugar blocking as a diet—more as just a means of getting the refined carbs *out* of her diet. "I used to eat a lot more sugar and starches," she said, but "cutting back on those went really easily. There were times when I had some [and] I felt like I was going overboard, but I still kept losing [weight]." The Sugar Blockers Diet also worked well for her because it consisted of eating! "I found it very easy to do, and I liked it. I think it's a 10, [with] 10 being the easiest. You can eat anything!"

after

3

THE DANGER
OF SUGAR
SHOCKS

O N THE REALITY TELEVISION show *The Biggest Loser,* you can watch overweight contestants starve themselves and put themselves through grueling exercise sessions to lose weight. Coaches browbeat the participants to get them to push the limits of their willpower.

I've been practicing medicine too long to place much stock in willpower when it comes to losing weight. People consistently overestimate their ability to control the amount of food they eat. They launch into a strict diet and stay on it for a while, but then their motivation wanes and they go back to their old ways.

If you're so powerless over your appetite, how can you lose weight? Actually, it's easier than you think.

People don't gain weight because they lack willpower. In most cases, the problem is that their bodies make too much insulin—up to five or six times the normal amounts. As you learned in the last chapter, excessive insulin locks calories in your fat stores so your body can't use them for energy. That's why, even though you have plenty of calories stored up as fat, you seem to be hungry all of the time. Too much insulin causes you to eat more calories than you burn off and makes it difficult for you to lose weight.

Here's the good news. You don't need to starve yourself to lose weight; you don't even need to reduce the amount of food you eat. You just need to reduce the amount of insulin your body makes. Of course, one way to do that would be to stop eating carbohydrates altogether. However, you don't have to go that far: You only have to cut out the carbs that are absorbed in your bloodstream too quickly—*the ones that cause after-meal blood sugar spikes.*

Just a minute—a carb is a carb, right? What difference does it make whether the carbs you eat are absorbed quickly or slowly?

● PUBLIC ENEMY NUMBER ONE: THE AFTER-MEAL SPIKE

Your beta cells' job is to keep your blood sugar in as narrow a range as possible. Within minutes of your eating a carbohydrate, your blood sugar begins to rise. The beta cells respond immediately by secreting insulin into your bloodstream. Insulin pushes sugar out of the blood and into various cells of your body. Blood sugar levels usually peak an hour or two after you eat carbohydrates and return to their baseline in 3 to 4 hours.

How high your blood sugar rises after you eat depends on how many carbohydrates you eat, how much insulin your beta cells make, and how sensitive your body is to insulin. But that's not all: It also depends on how fast glucose enters your bloodstream. Why? *It takes a lot more insulin to handle glucose that rushes into your bloodstream all at once than it does to handle the same amount of glucose that trickles in slowly.*

Imagine that a platoon of soldiers is defending a fort from an invading force. If the invaders attacked one by one, you wouldn't need many soldiers to fend them off. However, if they charged at once, you might need the whole battalion. The number of attackers might be the same, but the number of defenders needed to handle them depends on whether they charge all at once or little by little. That's how insulin works. You need more of it to handle sugar molecules that flood your bloodstream all at once than you do those that get absorbed more slowly.

If your diet is typical, most of the insulin you make is squandered on carbohydrates that are absorbed too quickly. All of those "invaders" are attacking at the same time. The key to reducing your body's demands for insulin is not necessarily to eliminate foods that break down into sugar but to *get sugar to trickle into your bloodstream slowly instead of rushing in all at once.*

How can you tell if too much sugar is rushing into your bloodstream too fast? People don't develop diabetes overnight. Their beta cells have trouble dealing with carbohydrates for years beforehand. During this "prediabetic" phase, your blood sugar levels are okay when you haven't eaten for a few hours, but they often go up higher than normal after you eat carbohydrates. That's why doctors do glucose tolerance tests to detect prediabetes. They measure your blood sugar after you consume a standard amount of glucose, looking for those glucose "spikes"—a warning sign for diabetes.

DIAGNOSING Diabetes and Prediabetes

DIAGNOSING DIABETES is pretty simple. Measure your blood sugar. If it's high, you've got it. If it's not, you don't. Doctors currently define diabetes as a fasting blood sugar level greater than 125 or a nonfasting blood sugar more than 200.

Doctors have learned to recognize people who are at increased risk of developing diabetes, a state they call prediabetes. People with prediabetes often have normal blood sugar levels when they are fasting, but because their beta cells are starting to fail, their blood sugar rises more than normal after they eat carbohydrates—after-meal "spikes."

The best way to tell if you're prediabetic is to check your blood sugar after you eat. You can actually do your own glucose tolerance test by measuring your blood sugar before and a couple of hours after you eat a starchy snack. Normally, it shouldn't rise more than 40 points. If

it does, you might have prediabetes, and you should talk to your doctor about it.

A doctor can tell if you're having sugar spikes even if you haven't had anything to eat for several hours. Every time your blood sugar spikes, even if it comes right back to normal, it puts a minuscule coat of sugar on the hemoglobin in your red blood cells, which stays there for up to 3 months.

Your doctor can measure the amount of sugar on your hemoglobin with a test called hemoglobin A1C. The level of hemoglobin A1C in your blood reflects your average blood sugar level over the previous 3 months. Many diabetics have near-normal *fasting* blood sugar levels but have high levels after meals, which raises their A1C level. Indeed, among treated diabetics, after-meal blood sugar surges account for as much as 70 percent of their abnormal blood sugar levels.

Blood sugar spikes are not just a sign of diabetes; they're also harmful to your arteries. Doctors now have monitoring devices they can attach to patients that record blood sugar levels continuously for several days at a time as patients go about their normal activities. This allows doctors to tell how much the blood sugar fluctuates from hour to hour. In a study reported in the *Journal of the American Medical Association,* French researchers estimated the amount of blood vessel damage that high blood sugar causes by measuring oxidized by-products of metabolism in the urine and compared it with the blood glucose fluctuations observed on continuous blood sugar monitoring. They found that after-meal blood sugar spikes caused more damage than did blood sugar levels that were continuously high.

● INSULIN SPIKES WITHOUT GLUCOSE SPIKES

Even if you're showing no signs of diabetes and your blood sugar levels are normal before and after meals, don't relax yet. Just because you don't have blood sugar spikes doesn't mean you're not having *insulin* spikes. Your body might be able to produce enough insulin to keep your blood sugar from rising too high—at least for now. But if you could measure how much insulin your body has to make to handle rapidly digested refined carbs, you would find that it's a lot more than if you ate only slowly digested ones, especially if you have insulin resistance. Indeed, excessive insulin production promotes weight gain, leads to high blood triglycerides and high blood pressure, and raises the risk of artery disease *even if you don't have diabetes.*

Refined carbohydrates seem to be especially harmful to women. Reporting in the *Archives of Internal Medicine,* Italian researchers analyzed the diets of 32,578 women without diabetes and tracked their health for 8 years. The women whose diets were highest in refined carbohydrates developed heart disease more than twice as often as women whose diets were lowest. There was no correlation with fat or cholesterol intake.

● GOOD CARBS AND BAD CARBS

There's no question that strict low-carbohydrate diets reduce blood sugar and insulin demands significantly. Swedish researchers found that patients with diabetes taking insulin who went on a low-carb diet were able to decrease their insulin doses from an average of 60 units to only 18 units per day. Some were able to discontinue insulin shots altogether.

If you eliminated carbohydrates from your diet, you would have no problems with after-meal blood sugar spikes. Reducing the amount of insulin in your system would allow calories to leave your fat stores and promote weight loss. Several studies have shown that people who follow low-carb diets *without trying to cut calories* actually consume fewer calories than do those on low-fat diets *who try to cut calories*. In fact, in the Swedish study mentioned above, subjects lost an average of 18 pounds and kept the weight off for 3 years after the study ended.

It's no surprise that avoiding carbohydrates reduces insulin demands. Your body hardly needs any insulin at all to handle other kinds of food—fat and protein. However, if you've ever tried a low-carbohydrate diet, you know that even though you can eat all the food you want, such diets are hard to stick with. They're easy to follow at first, but soon you start yearning for the missing foods. Fruits and vegetables contain vitamins, minerals, and fiber, which are essential to good health. Trying to eliminate all carbohydrates creates irresistible food cravings.

But if overproduction of insulin is the problem, and after-meal blood sugar spikes are what cause most insulin overproduction, what if you keep eating slowly digested carbs and just avoid the rapidly digested ones—the ones that cause after-meal glucose spikes? Indeed, you can get the benefits of a low-carb diet without depriving yourself of many of the foods you crave just by cutting out *refined* carbohydrates.

For example, in a study reported in 2007 in the *Journal of the American*

Medical Association, Boston researchers randomly assigned half of a group of overweight adults to a diet that allowed them to eat as much fat, protein, and fresh fruit and vegetables as they wanted but encouraged them to reduce their intake of rapidly digested refined carbohydrates such as bread, potatoes, and rice. The researchers assigned the other half to a low-fat, calorie-restricted diet. After 18 months, the subjects who just avoided refined carbohydrates *without trying to reduce their intake of other foods* lost more weight than did the participants following the low-fat diet *who were trying to reduce their food intake.*

Cutting out refined carbohydrates also has the same beneficial effects on cholesterol as following a strict low-carbohydrate diet: lower triglyceride levels and higher concentrations of good cholesterol. Bad-cholesterol levels usually stay the same or decrease slightly.

The advantage of cutting out rapidly digested "bad" carbs while continuing to eat slowly digested "good" carbs is that you get the same benefits as cutting out all carbs but without the irresistible food cravings. This is a style of eating (I won't call it a diet because it is so easy to follow) that people can stick to for life.

Sound simple? Well, as simple as avoiding refined carbohydrates is, these foods are staples of the modern diet. We're confronted with them at virtually every meal. It would be great if we could cut them out altogether, but sometimes they're hard to avoid.

But if glucose itself is not the problem—if it's just a matter of how fast carbs break down to glucose and enter your bloodstream—what if you could find a way to slow down the process, to make the glucose in refined carbohydrates trickle into your system slowly, like the glucose in fresh vegetables, instead of rushing in all at once?

Think it's a pipe dream? It can actually be done, and in fact, it *is* being done, and the results are remarkable.

4

THE POWER OF SUGAR BLOCKING

I F THE IDEA that you can lower your blood sugar by inhibiting the absorption of carbs once you eat them sounds too good to be true, consider the difference between broccoli and bread. A large serving of broccoli may release as much glucose into your bloodstream as a slice of bread would, but it won't raise your blood sugar as much. Why? Because broccoli contains substances that inhibit the absorption of glucose, and bread does not. Our food is full of natural sugar blockers. Although they don't actually stop carbs from being absorbed into the bloodstream, they slow the process.

Now here's what's cool: Some of those sugar blockers slow the absorption not only of the glucose in food that contains them *but also the glucose in other foods consumed with them*. You may wonder if all the carbs you eat eventually get absorbed anyway, what good it does just to delay the process. Well, the pharmaceutical industry has developed a medication called acarbose that can answer that question. It inhibits the breakdown of starch to sugar in the digestive tract similar to the natural sugar blockers in food. Because acarbose has no other known effects on the body—it doesn't even enter the bloodstream—it provides a good way to see what slowing carbohydrate digestion can do.

● STARCH BLOCKERS

If you haven't heard of acarbose, here's why. In the 1980s, with the obesity epidemic well under way, America was fertile ground for shortcuts to weight loss. Marketers of diet supplements started selling a product that they claimed stopped starch from being absorbed into the bloodstream. It was a powder made from white kidney beans that contained a substance called phaseolamin. Laboratory tests showed that phaseolamin could deactivate amylase, the intestinal enzyme responsible for breaking down starch to sugar. Supposedly, the supplement could keep you from absorbing some of the calories in starch so that you could continue eating your favorite carbs and still lose weight. Because phaseolamin was considered a natural food, marketers didn't need government approval to sell it and dieters didn't need a prescription to buy it.

It turned out that while phaseolamin worked in the test tube, it didn't do what it was supposed to in the body. The digestive tract is an inhospitable place for the substance. Stomach acid deactivates most of it before it reaches the small intestine, where the enzyme amylase does its work. Scientists found that taking phaseolamin made no difference in the amount of starch that was eventually absorbed into the bloodstream. Consequently, the government prohibited companies from marketing phaseolamin as a weight loss product, and it rapidly fell in popularity.

Unfortunately, America's experience with phaseolamin created skepticism toward the whole idea of sugar blocking. It became common wisdom that starch blockers, like other weight loss products that marketers were peddling, didn't work.

Nevertheless, the idea that a pill could inhibit starch from breaking down to glucose and being absorbed into the bloodstream was not as far-fetched as many people thought. Starch digestion depends on a single enzyme—amylase—which your pancreas secretes into your intestine when you eat. Scientists knew that if you could deactivate amylase, you would indeed keep starch from being absorbed into your bloodstream. So just as a lot of folks were wondering how they could have been so naive as to think that a pill could keep the food they ate from going into their system, the pharmaceutical industry introduced acarbose, a proven-effective amylase inhibitor that was approved by the FDA in 1999 for treating diabetes.

Acarbose works by mimicking starch. Like starch, it's made up of chains of sugar molecules linked end to end but in a slightly different pattern from that of starch. The difference is just enough that when amylase tries to break the links between acarbose's sugar molecules, as it does starch, it gets stuck. Acarbose takes amylase out of action. Tests show that taking acarbose before you eat a starch-containing meal reduces your after-meal blood sugar level by as much as 40 percent.

Unfortunately, acarbose came on the market about the same time that scientists were debunking the starch-blocking claims of phaseolamin. Consequently, the notion that a pill could inhibit starch absorption was viewed with skepticism. Besides, most doctors weren't worried much about carbohydrates. They were more concerned about fat and cholesterol. They figured, correctly, that if their patients were avoiding fat and cholesterol, they would probably be eating more starch, which meant that they would have to take acarbose several times a day. Acarbose's seemingly modest benefits didn't seem to be worth the trouble.

Another reason acarbose didn't gain much popularity among American doctors is that, while it does a good job lowering *after-meal* blood sugar levels, it has only minimal effects on *fasting* levels, which were the only ones doctors at that time paid attention to.

In the 1980s, the *New England Journal of Medicine* published the results of a study showing that while acarbose slows the digestion of starch, it doesn't actually keep it from ultimately being absorbed into the bloodstream. Most doctors at the time figured that it didn't make much difference if acarbose slowed the absorption of starch if it all ended up in the bloodstream anyway. They didn't pay much attention to after-meal blood sugar levels. The fact that the body needs less insulin to handle slowly absorbed carbs than it does rapidly absorbed ones hadn't been discovered yet.

The Surprising Benefits of Acarbose

In 2003, the *Journal of the American Medical Association* reported the results of a study called the STOP-NIDDM trial. In it, researchers followed 1,418 people with signs of early diabetes to see if acarbose could prevent them from developing full-fledged diabetes. They randomly treated half of the participants with acarbose and the other half with a placebo, a pill that looked like acarbose but contained no active ingredients. Acarbose proved useful not only for treating type 2 diabetes but also for keeping prediabetes from progressing to diabetes. After 4 years, there were 36 percent fewer new cases of diabetes among the subjects who took acarbose than among those who took the placebo.

That's impressive enough, but even more astonishing was acarbose's effects on the incidence of heart attacks. Acarbose reduced the heart attack rate by a mind-blowing *90 percent*. Most doctors found these results virtually unbelievable. They considered acarbose a diabetes drug, not a heart drug. It's a fair bet that most heart specialists didn't recognize it by name. Doctors had a hard time believing that a silly little pill like acarbose, which does nothing but slow starch absorption—it doesn't even enter the bloodstream—could prevent artery blockages. Most American doctors dismissed the STOP-NIDDM study as a fluke.

However, scientists later reviewed the results of every research study they could find that examined the effects of acarbose on the incidence of heart attacks and strokes. Indeed, their analysis, published in the *European Heart Journal,* confirmed that acarbose significantly reduced the incidence of heart attacks and strokes in patients with early type 2 diabetes or prediabetes.

When scientists started looking at acarbose's effects on risk factors for heart disease, including obesity, cholesterol imbalance, high blood pressure, and overactive blood clotting, the idea that acarbose could prevent heart attacks became more plausible. In addition to promoting weight loss and lowering blood sugar, acarbose improves the balance between good- and bad-cholesterol levels, reduces high blood pressure, and lowers the concentrations of blood clotting factors linked to heart attacks.

At the same time that scientists were discovering the benefits of acarbose, other scientists were discovering that diets full of natural substances that reduce after-meal blood sugar spikes had similar benefits. The notion that reducing after-meal blood sugar spikes prevents heart attacks was not so surprising after all.

Dietary Lessons from Acarbose

You may wonder whether the lower incidence of obesity, diabetes, and heart disease that researchers find among people who avoid refined carbohydrates is the result of factors other than reducing after-meal blood sugar surges. You could argue, for example, that the vitamins in the foods they eat to replace refined carbohydrates provide the benefits or that something besides glucose is the culprit behind those diseases. In fact, Americans consume most of their harmful trans fats in refined carbohydrates, so you may think that it's the trans fats in these foods that are the real problem.

Acarbose provides an ideal way to study the effects of reducing after-meal blood sugar spikes without otherwise altering the diet—indeed, without even reducing carbohydrate intake. Taking acarbose without making any other changes in the diet brings the same benefits that researchers have associated with low-carb diets: weight loss, lower blood sugar, reduced insulin needs, a lower risk of diabetes, lower triglyceride levels, and higher concentrations of good cholesterol. Acarbose provides proof that not all carbs have equal effects on blood sugar and that reducing the speed with which carbs enter the bloodstream can have significant benefits.

It might seem hard to believe that such a simple thing as blunting blood sugar spikes—not even preventing them—could have such benefits, but if you consider what scientists now know about carbohydrate metabolism, it makes perfect sense. When it comes to producing excessive amounts of insulin, the problem is not food in general—your body doesn't need insulin to handle fat and protein. The problem is, indeed, carbohydrates, but not all carbohydrates. The culprits are the foods that rush into your bloodstream quickly instead of slowly. As it turns out, the substance in our diet that is responsible for most blood sugar spikes is starch. Considering that starch digestion is entirely dependent on a single enzyme, it's not surprising that even modest inhibition of that enzyme's action would have beneficial effects.

● SUGAR BLOCKERS: A SPECIAL ROLE IN TREATING DIABETES

Doctors have effective medications for reducing *fasting* blood sugar levels. However, they don't have many drugs for blunting after-meal blood sugar spikes. And while most diabetes medications, including insulin, are good at preventing the damage to small blood vessels that harms the eyes, kidneys, and nerves, they're not as effective against the damage to large blood vessels that leads to heart disease and strokes. That's where sugar blockers, whether in natural food or medications, come in. As research studies on acarbose show, it takes surprisingly little inhibition of glucose absorption to lower insulin demands, decrease blood sugar, improve cholesterol balance, thwart progression to diabetes, and reduce the risk of heart disease.

Sugar blockers also have a role in preventing prediabetes from tipping into full-blown type 2 diabetes. After-meal blood sugar spikes create most of the excessive demands for insulin that wear out your beta cells and lead to diabetes. As shown by the STOP-NIDDM study, slowing the absorption of carbohydrates prevents progression to diabetes and can actually reverse prediabetes.

● NATURAL SUGAR BLOCKERS

Now that you know what acarbose can do, imagine getting similar results by natural means—without taking a pill. Many foods and natural supplements inhibit glucose absorption and reduce insulin demands as effectively as medications like acarbose do.

Your digestive tract has to break down the foods you eat to their basic building blocks—amino acids, fatty acids, and glucose—before they can be absorbed into your bloodstream. The time it takes for this to occur is, in a sense, a natural regulator of the speed with which nutrients enter your system. The problem is that our digestive tracts were designed for the Stone Age—made to handle food that was much harder to digest than the food we eat now. Most carbohydrates in their natural form contain inhibitors to digestion—structures and substances that interfere with the breakdown and absorption of starch and sugar. It takes hours for the digestive tract to break down fresh vegetation to glucose and absorb it into the bloodstream. Our intestines evolved to be powerful extractors of glucose from unrefined vegetation, such as roots, bark, grasses, and unripe fruits and vegetables.

However, when carbohydrates are altered, or "refined," by humans, they lose their natural sugar blockers. Compared with what our ancestors ate in prehistoric times, many of the carbohydrates we eat now—particularly starchy staples like bread, potatoes, and rice—are ridiculously easy to digest. Whereas other foods require the entire 22 feet of the small intestine to be digested, starch and sugar get absorbed *in the first few inches*. This super-rapid absorption of refined carbohydrates creates a mismatch between the intestine's ability to absorb glucose and the body's capacity to handle it.

Acarbose and other sugar blockers restore, to some degree, a more natural balance between the kinds of carbohydrates we eat and the speed with which our digestive system breaks them down and absorbs them.

You can be assured that no matter what kind of sugar blocker you use, your digestive tract will win in the end. Everything you eat that is digestible *will* get digested. Indeed, if you look at the research on sugar blockers, you might not be impressed by how much a particular blocker lowers blood sugar. Acarbose, which is considered a highly effective sugar blocker, may reduce after-meal blood sugar spikes by only 30 percent. That might not seem like much—you'd probably prefer no spike at all—but remember, it doesn't take much sugar blocking to make a big difference when it comes to reducing insulin demands, preventing diabetes, improving cholesterol balance, and lowering heart attack risk.

● A CARBOHYDRATE'S JOURNEY

Changes at any step that carbohydrates take in their journey from your lips to the cells in your body can raise or lower your blood sugar. To get a better understanding of the steps in the digestive process where sugar blockers can work, let's follow a carb—say, a forkful of spaghetti—as it travels from your lips to the cells in your body, where it's used for energy or stored as fat.

The Grinder

The first step in carbohydrate digestion is mastication, the process of chewing. The smaller those spaghetti particles are when they reach your stomach, the faster you'll digest them. That's why thin, stringy pasta, such as angel-hair pasta, will raise your blood sugar more than pasta made of larger noodles, such as lasagna. Also, if you prepare your pasta al dente, or slightly undercooked, so it's more chunky when you swallow it, it will take longer to digest and raise your blood sugar less than if you overcook it.

The Holding Bin

The next stop is your stomach. Food does not get absorbed there. Rather, your stomach acts as a hopper—a holding bin and a regulator of the speed with which food passes into the small intestine, where it is absorbed into your bloodstream. If your stomach already contains food, the spaghetti will have to wait its turn before it can continue its journey. Carbs consumed on a full stomach raise your blood sugar less than do carbs consumed on an empty stomach. If you eat a bulky low–glycemic load food, such as a salad with lots of raw vegetables, before you eat the spaghetti, it will delay its absorption and reduce your after-meal blood sugar level.

The Control Valve

At the outlet of your stomach is a muscular ring, the pyloric valve. It regulates the speed with which food leaves your stomach and enters the small intestine. Hormones and nerve circuits that originate in centers farther down your intestine control your pyloric valve. This arrangement comprises a feedback system to prevent food from passing too quickly through your system. When your intestine senses that more food is traveling through it than it can handle, it sends the message to the pyloric valve to tighten up and slow the passage of food.

Starch is so easy to digest that once it gets into your intestine, there's little to keep it from being absorbed. Your pyloric valve is all that stands between the spaghetti in your stomach and a surge of glucose in your bloodstream. Will your pyloric valve get the message to slow down? Maybe, maybe not. Whereas other foods travel most of the 22-foot length of your small intestine as they are being digested, that spaghetti probably won't make it 2 feet before it is absorbed into your bloodstream. Most of it won't reach the centers farther along that send feedback messages to your pyloric valve.

However, you can get your intestine to tell the pyloric valve to slow down by eating food that sends the message before you eat the spaghetti. The most potent inhibitor of stomach emptying is fat. When just a little fat—a couple of teaspoons—reaches your intestine, it activates a reflex that slows the passage of food through your pyloric valve. If you eat a fatty snack—a handful of nuts, a piece of cheese, or a pork rind—a few minutes before eating the spaghetti, it will reduce your after-meal blood sugar surge.

The Splitters

Once the spaghetti reaches your intestine, there's one more step it has to take before it can enter your bloodstream. It must be broken down to its basic building block: glucose. Starch consists of long chains of glucose molecules linked end to end, like railroad cars. Your digestive tract has to split them apart before they can be absorbed into the bloodstream, and there's only one enzyme that can do it—amylase. Amylase unhitches the glucose molecules and frees them up so that they can be absorbed. Without amylase, the spaghetti would go right through your digestive tract and out in your stool. Your weight problems would be over, and your type 2 diabetes would be cured!

But that won't happen. Your pancreas makes plenty of amylase—way more than you need. Remember, your digestive tract was designed to handle carbohydrates that are much harder to digest than spaghetti—things like roots and bark. Pitting all that amylase against those starch molecules is like sending a battalion of Marines out to round up a gang of kindergartners. By putting amylase into better balance with starch, amylase inhibitors such as acarbose level the playing field. They make starch behave more like fresh fruits and vegetables so that glucose trickles into your bloodstream slowly instead of rushing in all at once. Many plants contain amylase inhibitors; their purpose is to protect plants from being devoured by insects and bacteria. And some natural foods have effects similar to acarbose. Vinegar, for example, inhibits amylase and lowers after-meal blood sugar levels.

Sponges

After the glucose molecules in the spaghetti are unhitched from one another, they float around in solution in your digestive juices until they come in contact with the walls of your intestine, where tiny "transporters" latch onto them and pull them into your bloodstream. You can slow the absorption of glucose by eating foods that soak up intestinal juices and keep dissolved glucose from coming in contact with your intestinal lining. In Chapter 6 you will learn about foods and supplements that contain an indigestible kind of carbohydrate, called soluble fiber, that absorbs glucose molecules and prevents them from getting near those transporters—one of nature's ways of keeping glucose from rushing into your bloodstream.

The Shock Absorber

Once glucose gets into the blood that flows to your intestine, it has one more stop before it reaches the rest of your body: the liver. Your liver largely determines the composition of your blood, removing things that might be harmful and adding things the body needs. One of the liver's jobs is to keep your blood sugar from rising too high after you eat—it acts as sort of a sugar "shock absorber." Your liver removes glucose from your blood after you eat—an action that is helped by insulin—and adds glucose back to your blood when you haven't eaten for a while. This shock-absorber function is one of the first things to go haywire when you start heading toward diabetes.

Some of the most effective medicines for diabetes act by helping the liver take up glucose after you eat and keeping it from releasing glucose into the blood when it shouldn't. Such medicines not only lower blood sugar but also promote weight loss and can actually prevent diabetes. Several natural substances can also help the liver take up glucose after you eat—for example, a shot of alcohol or a fatty snack taken before a meal.

First Responders

Once out of your liver, blood from your digestive tract mixes with blood coming from the rest of your body. Your heart then pumps it to all parts of your body, including the beta cells of your pancreas. These sense your blood sugar rising and respond by secreting insulin to lower it.

How effective insulin is at lowering your after-meal blood sugar has a lot to do with timing. The sooner your beta cells secrete insulin into your bloodstream after you eat a carbohydrate, the less insulin you will need to lower your blood sugar. It's like a fire department responding to a fire. The sooner the alarm goes off, the fewer firefighters will be needed to put out the fire.

Your beta cells have a special supply of insulin ready to be released at the first sign of the spaghetti heading toward your bloodstream. Just having food in your intestine, even before the spaghetti enters your bloodstream, will prompt the beta cells to release this cache of insulin into your bloodstream. This is called the first-phase insulin response. Because this burst of insulin occurs so quickly, it keeps your blood sugar from rising as much as it would otherwise and reduces the total amount of insulin you need to handle a meal.

There are several ways you can enhance the first-phase insulin response. Protein triggers a first-phase response even though it contains no glucose. For example, if you have a meatball with your spaghetti, it will increase the first-phase response and reduce the size of your after-meal blood sugar surge.

The Order-and-Delivery System

The composition of your blood is the same everywhere in your body. However, the needs of different cells vary. The composition of the fluid in each cell must be carefully and individually controlled; otherwise the cell will malfunction or even die. Indeed, if glucose were allowed to flow freely into cells, it would kill them. That doesn't happen because every cell in your body is surrounded by a membrane that regulates the flow of substances into and out of it. When a cell needs a delivery of glucose, it sends glucose transporters to the membrane surface, where they pluck glucose molecules from the blood and pull them into the cell. Although insulin is necessary to activate the transporters, if a cell has all the glucose it needs, it stops producing transporters. Even if the blood that bathes the cell contains plenty of insulin, it won't take up glucose—it becomes "insulin resistant."

So the last part of your spaghetti's journey is to get across those cell membranes. Your muscle cells are by far the biggest users of glucose and the target of most of the insulin you make. The reason you become insulin resistant is that your muscles become resistant. They stop making glucose transporters, and the only good way to get them to start making transporters again is to exercise them. When you exercise your muscles, each muscle cell you use switches on the production of glucose transporters, which pull glucose out of your bloodstream and into the cell. These glucose transporters stay on the cell membrane for 24 hours or so, then start diminishing. As long as you exercise your muscles every 24 to 48 hours, they will stay sensitive to insulin.

A Relief Valve

There's another way to get your muscles to remove glucose from your blood that is independent of insulin. Normally, when you exercise, it takes a few hours for your muscle cells to make glucose transporters and start responding to insulin. This presents a problem: If your muscle cells are going to use glucose as fuel, they will need it as soon as you start exercising, not in a few hours. Your body has a way of solving this problem. Activating your muscles instantly opens up special channels in your muscle-cell membranes that are independent of insulin. Glucose flows into your muscle cells as soon as you start exercising and stops when you stop. Thus, one of the best ways to reduce an after-meal blood sugar spike is to get up and engage in gentle exercise soon after eating.

Blocking Sugar at Several Steps

You see, then, that you can inhibit the breakdown of carbohydrates to glucose and its entry into your bloodstream at several points in the journey from your lips to the cells of your body. How high your blood sugar rises after a meal is not simply a matter of how much carbohydrate you eat or how much insulin you make. To summarize, here is a list of the ways that you can blunt after-meal blood sugar spikes according to the parts of the digestive process that each affects.

► **Particle-size increasers:** Ways to increase the size of carbohydrate particles that reach your stomach.
Example: Preparing pasta al dente to make it crunchy.

► **Stomach barriers:** Things you can do to physically impede the passage of carbohydrates from your stomach to your intestine.
Example: Starting your meal with a salad.

- **Intestinal "brakes":** Substances that activate normal reflexes that arise from the intestine and slow stomach emptying.
  Example: Eating a handful of nuts before a meal.

- **Enzyme inhibitors:** Substances that inhibit enzymes that break down starch to sugar.
  Example: Vinegar (as in a salad dressing).

- **Sugar sponges:** Substances that soak up glucose in your digestive tract and prevent it from coming in contact with your intestinal lining, where it is absorbed.
  Example: High-fiber foods or supplements.

- **Liver helpers:** Substances that enhance your liver's ability to take up glucose released into your bloodstream during meals.
  Example: A glass of wine with your meal.

- **First-phase stimulators:** Ways to get your beta cells to secrete insulin sooner rather than later after you eat carbohydrates, which makes insulin more effective.
  Example: Eating an egg with your toast.

- **Insulin sensitizers:** Techniques that sensitize your body to insulin so that less is needed to handle after-meal glucose surges.
  Example: Exercising every 24 to 48 hours.

- **After-meal exercise:** Taking advantage of your muscles' ability to remove sugar from your bloodstream without insulin.
  Example: Taking a walk after a meal.

● THE POWER OF COMBINING SUGAR BLOCKERS

An especially effective technique is to combine sugar blockers that work on different parts of your digestive system. For example, researchers found that combining a "sponge" type of sugar blocker, such as soluble fiber, with an enzyme inhibitor, such as vinegar, lowers after-meal blood sugar more than doubling the amount of either sugar blocker alone. Similarly, the most effective sugar-blocking medications are those that act on several steps in the digestive process. In Chapter 13 you'll learn about a new class of medication called GLP-1 analogs that block sugar at several different parts of the digestive process at once. Not only do these reduce after-meal blood sugar and insulin levels, but they also produce significant and lasting weight loss.

In the chapters to come, you will see that sugar blocking is not just about food or medication. It's about the whole context in which you eat your meals—the activities that surround meals, including whether you have exercised, how relaxed you are, and how much sleep you get. The more of these things you have working in your favor, the more successful you will be at controlling your blood sugar and your body's insulin demands.

Of course, you don't need a sugar blocker for a meal that contains no refined carbohydrates, such as a salad or an omelet. You don't even need one for a meal that contains carbohydrates that trickle into your bloodstream slowly, as many fruits and vegetables do. You need sugar blockers only for the carbs that cause sugar shocks. How will you recognize the culprits when you see them?

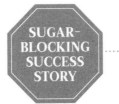
Age: 61

Height: 5' 4"

Pounds lost: 12

Inches lost: 5¼

Major accomplishment:
Reduced triglyceride levels by more than half!

Favorite sugar blockers:
Walnuts, almonds, and olive oil

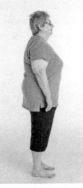

before

SANDI HAUSMAN
Strength in Sugar Blocking

SANDI HAUSMAN started the Sugar Blockers Diet as a self-declared carb–and cola addict. In the past, it was easy for her to make excuses for a few guilty pleasures—especially as someone who was in good health and took daily vitamins. But once Sandi hit 60, she realized that her weight was starting to hold her back. More and more aches were creeping up in her feet, knees, and hips, and her "numbers" (cholesterol, blood sugar, blood pressure), while they weren't warranting any medications, were high enough to alarm her.

Fast-forward a few weeks on the Sugar Blockers Diet, and Sandi isn't able to stomach even the thought of a Coke. "In the past I could never give it up," she said. But once she understood the negative effects that soda has on the body—specifically blood sugar—it was easy to give it up. And those aches and pains? Gone.

"My weight had always been an issue," said Sandi, who had breast cancer 15 years ago. "But my second chemo treatment threw me into early menopause, and I gained [an extra] 45 pounds." After successfully battling breast cancer, Sandi knew she could beat the weight gain, and she also wanted to start making changes for an overall healthier lifestyle. With a 12-pound weight loss in her 6 weeks on the plan (and an additional 14 pounds in the next 6 weeks), she's well on her way.

"I go to work every day and take a little container of walnuts," Sandi said. "Beats a Tasty Kake!" Not to mention, using sugar blockers has helped keep her postmeal blood sugar spikes on an even keel. As a prime example, there were many days when Sandi would have a low blood sugar count after a relatively carb-free meal of meatballs with salad and dressing, but the next night—after she ate meat loaf with some mashed potatoes—her blood sugar was the same as the previous count! Why? Because she'd had a salad with a vinegar-based dressing 20 minutes before enjoying a little bit of starch. Turns out you can have your cake (or potatoes, as the case may be) and eat it too!

Sandi plans to stick with these healthy habits she's developed . . . mostly because it's so easy to do. She loves that the Sugar Blockers Diet is a natural fit with food planning, especially compared with other weight loss programs she's tried. On those, "you always need to figure out points and portion sizes," she said. But now "there's nothing off-limits. We're going out with friends on Friday night, and we're looking forward to that. I just know what I need to do before I go." In fact, Sandi's husband, who does the cooking and has become more creative in adding sugar-blocking ingredients like olive oil and almonds to the menu, has also lost about 6 pounds.

And co-workers have noticed not just her weight but also her "new" wardrobe—discovered in her very own closet. "I haven't worn these pants in about 10 years," said a smiling Sandi. "I'll gladly retire what I bought last year!"

after

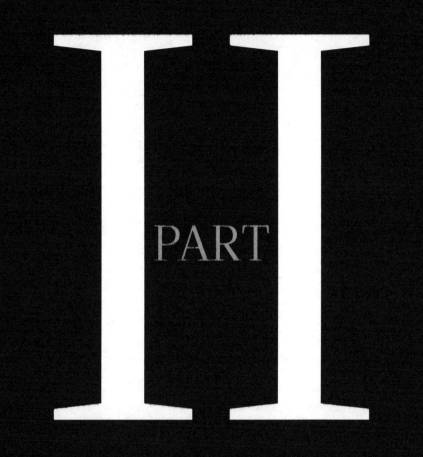

PART II

SUGAR BLOCKERS
FOR SUGAR SHOCKERS

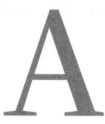S YOU LEARNED IN PART I, you can take measures at several steps in the digestive process to slow the absorption of glucose into your bloodstream. In Part II you'll learn to recognize the foods that cause blood sugar spikes and the foods that blunt those spikes.

Of course, you don't need sugar blockers for meals that won't raise your blood sugar. Chances are most of your favorite foods hardly raise blood sugar at all. You will see that there are only a handful of culprits. However, while few in number, these foods aren't just a little worse than other foods; they're *much* worse. You need to be able to recognize them on sight.

The next chapter will give you a sharp eye for distinguishing between foods you can enjoy freely and those you need to limit or block. The following chapters show you how to put Mother Nature's sugar blockers to work to reduce the harmful effects of those culprits when they do sneak into your diet.

5

IDENTIFYING THE CULPRITS

FOR YEARS, doctors thought that when it came to blood sugar, it didn't matter whether you consumed carbohydrates in the form of broccoli, bread, or chocolate. They figured the only thing that mattered was how much glucose a carbohydrate eventually released into your bloodstream. They knew that the fiber in fruits and vegetables was indigestible but figured that the remainder, the so-called "available carbohydrate," raised blood sugar the same, regardless of what food it came from.

However, nobody actually systematically measured the effects of various carbohydrates on blood glucose levels. It wasn't until the 1980s that the assumption that "a carb is a carb" was tested. Researchers at the University of Toronto, led by Dr. David Jenkins, conducted hundreds of experiments in which they had subjects consume identical amounts of available carbohydrate in different foods, and afterward measured blood sugar and insulin levels. What they found surprised them. They learned that it's difficult to predict from carbohydrate content alone how much a particular food will raise blood sugar. It's not as simple as "a carb is a carb." For example, a given amount of available carbohydrate consumed in the form of a baked potato raises blood sugar twice as much as the same amount of available carbohydrate consumed in the form of sliced peaches. Most surprising was that some carbohydrates—white bread, for instance—raise blood sugar *as much as pure sugar does.*

The Toronto researchers expressed the blood sugar–raising effects of different foods as the percentage that 50 grams of available carbohydrate in a food raises blood sugar compared with 50 grams of pure glucose. For example, they assigned an apple a value of 39 because 50 grams of available carbohydrate in an apple raises blood sugar 39 percent as much as 50 grams of pure glucose do. They called these measurements *glycemic indexes.*

● GLYCEMIC LOAD: A MORE PRACTICAL TOOL

The scientists who developed the glycemic indexes were trying to prove a point: that some foods raise blood sugar more than others do, even if they eventually release the same amount of glucose into the bloodstream. They didn't intend for their measurements to be used as an eating guide. Nevertheless, several diet-book authors seized on the glycemic indexes as a way for low-carb dieters to eat some carbohydrates and still lose weight.

However, there's a problem with using the glycemic indexes as a guide to eating. These are raw laboratory measurements. The amounts of food that the researchers gave subjects in order to measure effects on blood sugar—50 grams of available carbohydrate—bore no relationship to the amounts that people typically eat.

Consequently, scientists at Harvard University developed a method of predicting the blood sugar–raising effects of various foods that people can actually use as a guide to eating. Called the *glycemic load,* it represents the amount that a typical serving of a food (not necessarily 50 grams) raises blood sugar. To be practical, they used a single slice of white bread

HOW I CALCULATE Glycemic Load

I MADE A SLIGHT CHANGE in my glycemic load lists from other published listings to make them more user-friendly. To convert the glycemic load values you see on other listings so that they're comparable to the ones I use throughout this book, simply multiply those values by 10. For example, in the International Table of Glycemic Index and Glycemic Load Values, the glycemic load value for angel food cake is 19; on my list it would be 190. I did this so that a slice of white bread would turn out to have a glycemic load of 100. That way, the glycemic loads of various foods can be regarded as percentages of the glycemic load of a slice of white bread. For instance, if an apple has a glycemic load of 78, that means it would raise your blood sugar 78 percent as much as a slice of white bread would.

GLYCEMIC INDEX VERSUS Glycemic Load

AVAILABLE CARBOHYDRATE is the total amount of carbohydrate a food contains minus indigestible fiber. It represents the carbohydrate that eventually enters your bloodstream. The glycemic index reflects the blood sugar–raising effects of 50 grams of available carbohydrate in a food compared with 50 grams of pure glucose.

As important as the glycemic index research was, it led to some misleading conclusions. Make no mistake: A serving of pasta at your local Italian restaurant will raise your blood sugar more than a carrot will, but the glycemic index of a carrot is 49, and that of spaghetti is 46. What's wrong with this picture?

The problem is that carrots contain a lot of indigestible fiber and water and not much available carbohydrate. To get 50 grams of available carbohydrate, the researchers had to feed subjects seven full-size carrots. Who eats that many carrots at once?

The glycemic *load* refers to the blood sugar–raising effects of amounts of food that *people typically eat*. A typical serving of carrot—one carrot—has a glycemic load of 7. A restaurant-size serving of spaghetti—2 cups—has a glycemic load of 276. The glycemic loads more accurately reflect what foods do to your blood sugar in real life.

as the standard. For instance, a pear has a glycemic load of 57, which means that eating a typical-size pear raises blood sugar 57 percent as much as eating a slice of white bread.

In 2002, the *American Journal of Clinical Nutrition* published a list of glycemic loads titled the International Table of Glycemic Index and Glycemic Load Values, which became a common reference for physicians and nutritionists. The table on the next page, lists the glycemic loads of a few common foods. You can see, for example, that the glycemic loads of the fruit and vegetables are lower than those of the refined carbohydrates. Appendix C contains a list of the glycemic loads of more than 200 foods.

Glycemic Loads of Common Foods

FOOD	SERVING SIZE	GLYCEMIC LOAD (PERCENT OF 1 SLICE OF WHITE BREAD)
Carrot	1 medium	7
Tomato	1 medium	14
Apple	1 medium	78
White bread	1 slice	100
Spaghetti	2 cups	276
Bagel	1 medium	340

The glycemic load calculations produced valuable insights into the effects of various kinds of foods on health. Researchers found that diets containing large amounts of high-glycemic load foods raise the risk not only of diabetes and obesity but also of heart disease, menstrual disorders, age-related vision loss, acne, and some types of cancer.

Most helpfully, the glycemic load measurements provide a framework for a way of eating that allows you to enjoy the largest-possible variety of carbohydrates with the least impact on your blood sugar and insulin demands. Indeed, the best way to reduce your body's needs for insulin, short of avoiding carbohydrates altogether, is to take advantage of the natural sugar-blocking structures and substances in carbohydrates to reduce the glycemic load of your meals.

What's remarkable about the glycemic load measurements is how seemingly modest changes in diet can produce dramatic changes in glycemic load. In the table on the next page, compare a typical day's menu for a person not paying attention to glycemic load with that of a person eating just as heartily but consuming foods with lower glycemic loads. Notice how well you can eat and yet end up with a glycemic load that's a fraction of what it would be if you weren't trying to avoid high-glycemic load foods.

Low–Glycemic Load Pattern versus Typical Eating Pattern

LOW-GLYCEMIC LOAD PATTERN		TYPICAL PATTERN	
FOOD	GLYCEMIC LOAD	FOOD	GLYCEMIC LOAD
BREAKFAST			
Bacon	0	Orange juice	68
Eggs	0	Bagel	340
Coffee	0	Coffee	0
Sugar 1 tsp	28	Sugar 1 tsp	28
SNACK			
Latte	27	Coffee	0
Apple	78	Sugar 1 tsp	28
		Doughnut	205
LUNCH			
Chicken Caesar salad (no croutons)	0	Turkey sandwich	260
Milk	27	Potato chips	77
		Coca-Cola	218
SNACK			
Mixed nuts	7	Corn chips	97
DINNER			
Green salad	0	Caesar salad (with croutons)	100
12-oz steak	0	Spaghetti (2 cups)	276
Mushrooms	0	French bread	284
Asparagus	0	Butter	0
⅓ baked potato	82	Red wine	0
Butter	0	Cookie	114
Sour cream	0		
Dark chocolate	68		
Total glycemic load	**317**	**Total glycemic load**	**2,095**

What's a healthy glycemic load? The Nurses' Health Study, a study of the diets of more than 100,000 American women, found that the risk of diabetes, obesity, and heart disease begins to increase when the average daily glycemic load exceeds approximately 500. That's also the point below which natural weight loss occurs in overweight individuals with insulin resistance or type 2 diabetes.

● THE CULPRIT

One way that you could keep track of the glycemic load of your diet would be to add up the glycemic loads of the different foods you eat as you go through the day. However, there's a much simpler way to keep your glycemic load where it needs to be. Take a good look at the table below. This is a list of the glycemic loads of common foods that Americans eat, arranged in descending order so that the foods with the highest glycemic loads are at the top of the list and those with the lowest are at the bottom. Remember that the glycemic load is the percentage that a typical serving of food raises blood sugar in comparison with a slice of white bread. In this list, instead of specifying *units* of food, such as 1 slice of bread or 1 cup of macaroni, I used amounts that people commonly eat. For example, people usually eat 2 slices of bread when they have a sandwich or 2 cups of pasta when it's the main dish.

Glycemic Loads of Common Foods in Descending Order

FOOD	DESCRIPTION	TYPICAL SERVING	GLYCEMIC LOAD (PERCENTAGE OF 1 SLICE OF WHITE BREAD)
Pancake	5" diameter	2¹/₂ oz	346
Bagel	1 medium	3¹/₃ oz	340
Orange soda	12-oz can	12 oz	314
Macaroni	2 cups	10 oz	301

(continued)

Glycemic Loads of Common Foods
in Descending Order *(cont.)*

FOOD	DESCRIPTION	TYPICAL SERVING	GLYCEMIC LOAD (PERCENTAGE OF 1 SLICE OF WHITE BREAD)
White rice	1 cup	6^1/$_2$ oz	283
Spaghetti	2 cups	10 oz	276
White bread	2 slices, ^{3}/$_8$" thick	2^3/$_4$ oz	260
Baked potato	1 medium	5 oz	246
Whole wheat bread	2 slices, ^{3}/$_8$" thick	2^3/$_4$ oz	234
Raisin bran	1 cup	2 oz	227
Brown rice	1 cup	6^1/$_2$ oz	222
French fries	Medium serving (McDonald's)	5^1/$_4$ oz	219
Coca-Cola	12-oz can	12 oz	218
Hamburger bun	Top and bottom, 5" diameter	2^1/$_2$ oz	213
English muffin	1 medium	2 oz	208
Doughnut	1 medium	2 oz	205
Cornflakes	1 cup	1 oz	199
Corn on the cob	1 ear	5^1/$_3$ oz	171
Blueberry muffin	2^1/$_2$" diameter	2 oz	169
Instant oatmeal (cooked)	1 cup	8 oz	154
Chocolate cake	1 slice (4" × 4" × 1")	3 oz	154
Grape-Nuts	1 cup	1 oz	142
Cheerios	1 cup	1 oz	142
Special K	1 cup	1oz	133
Cookie	1 medium	1 oz	114
White bread (laboratory standard)	**1 slice (4" × ^{1}/$_4$")**	**1^1/$_{16}$ oz**	**100**
Tortilla (corn)	1 medium	1^1/$_4$ oz	85
Banana	1 medium	3^1/$_4$ oz	85
All-Bran	^{1}/$_2$ cup	1 oz	85
Tortilla (wheat)	1 medium	1^3/$_4$ oz	80

FOOD	DESCRIPTION	TYPICAL SERVING	GLYCEMIC LOAD (PERCENTAGE OF 1 SLICE OF WHITE BREAD)
Apple	1 medium	5½ oz	78
Grapefruit juice (unsweetened)	6 oz	6 oz	75
Orange	1 medium	6 oz	71
Pinto beans	½ cup	3 oz	57
Pear	1 medium	6 oz	57
Pineapple	1 slice (¾" × 3½" wide)	3 oz	50
Peach	1 medium	4 oz	47
Grapes	1 cup (40 grapes)	2½ oz	47
Kidney beans	½ cup	3 oz	40
Grapefruit	½	4½ oz	32
Table sugar	1 round tsp	⅙ oz	28
Milk (whole)	8 oz	8 oz	27
Peas	¼ cup	1½ oz	16
Tomato	1 medium	5 oz	15
Strawberries	1 cup	5½ oz	13
Carrot (raw)	1 medium (7½")	3 oz	11
Peanuts	¼ cup	1¼ oz	7
Spinach	1 cup	2½ oz	0
Pork	Two 5-oz chops	10 oz	0
Margarine	Typical serving	¼ oz	0
Lettuce	1 cup	2½ oz	0
Fish	8-oz fillet	8 oz	0
Eggs	1 egg	1½ oz	0
Cucumber	1 cup	6 oz	0
Chicken	1 breast	10 oz	0
Cheese	1 slice (2" × 2" × 1")	2 oz	0
Butter	1 tablespoon	¼ oz	0
Broccoli	½ cup	1½ oz	0
Beef	10-oz steak	10 oz	0

Now notice that, with the exception of soft drinks, *virtually every food with a glycemic load of more than 100 is a starch.* Also notice that almost every fruit and vegetable has a glycemic load of less than 100. Fruits and vegetables are carbohydrates, too, and they raise blood sugar a little but nothing compared with starches.

Here's the take-home lesson: Starches aren't just a little worse than fruits and vegetables; *they're terrible.* You'd have to gobble up seven peaches to match the glycemic load of a bagel or choke down 10 cups of peanuts to equal the glycemic load of a serving of spaghetti.

The reality is that, for most of us, fruits and vegetables in their natural state—so-called unrefined carbohydrates—don't raise blood sugar and insulin demands enough to worry about. They contain natural sugar-blocking structures and substances that slow the absorption of glucose into the bloodstream. The only carbs you need to avoid are ones that humans have *refined*—separated from their natural sugar-blocking constituents. This includes whole grain versions of starches, such as brown rice and whole wheat bread. The good news is that only a handful of carbs fall into this category. Here are some of the most common culprits.

- White bread
- Whole wheat bread
- White rice
- Brown rice
- Potatoes
- Corn
- Pasta
- Breakfast cereals

- Oatmeal
- Pancakes
- Bagels
- English muffins
- Cookies
- Crackers
- Potato chips
- Cornbread

Got the message? Anything made from potatoes, rice, corn, wheat, and other grains is a starch. Get rid of as many as you can. According to the

Nurses' Health Study, the total glycemic loads from these foods among Americans are more than 20 times that of any other food, including candy. They're mostly starch, and starch is nothing but a bunch of sugar molecules laid end to end. Those mashed potatoes you had last night? You might as well have eaten a pile of sugar. As soon as starch reaches your small intestine, it melts like a snowball in hot water, turns to sugar, and within a few minutes is in your bloodstream.

Starch contains no vital nutrients. You can only benefit by getting rid of it. The best thing you can do for weight problems or diabetes is not to worry

Gluten

GLUTEN IS a protein present in small amounts in many grains, including wheat. Some people have a kind of allergy to gluten called gluten intolerance, or celiac disease, which causes them to develop antibodies that damage normal tissues. Sufferers often develop severe health problems, including chronic diarrhea, an inability to absorb nutrients, anemia, weight loss, bone deterioration, and mysterious abdominal pains.

Gluten intolerance can usually be diagnosed with a blood test, although sometimes an intestinal biopsy is required. The treatment is to abstain from eating gluten-containing foods, mainly wheat products. It takes several weeks of avoiding gluten before symptoms resolve.

Although not a rare disease, gluten intolerance is uncommon, affecting less than 1 percent of the population. Thanks to stories in the media about sufferers whose disease went undiagnosed for years, many people these days who do not have gluten intolerance think they have the condition and seem to feel better when they avoid gluten-containing foods. Indeed, if you eliminate wheat products, you get rid of a major source of starch. Eliminating gluten-containing foods is harmless enough, unless you come to believe that gluten-free starches, such as potatoes, corn, and rice, are somehow good for you. Starch will raise your blood sugar whether it contains gluten or not.

about eggs, meat, dairy products, nuts, or fresh fruits and vegetables. Instead, just concentrate on limiting refined carbohydrates.

Now, here's how you can control your glycemic load each day without having to add up the glycemic loads of all the foods you eat. If you're typical, the glycemic loads of the *nonstarchy* carbohydrates you eat in an average day—salads, vegetables, fruit, etc.—don't add up to more than 250. As you see in the tables, the glycemic load of a typical serving of starch averages around 250. So here's a simple rule that will practically guarantee that your daily glycemic load won't exceed 500: *Don't eat more than the equivalent of one serving of starch a day.* That means you can eat a third of a serving three times a day, a half serving twice a day, or a full serving once a day. Just make sure the total is less than one serving of starch a day.

A lifetime eating plan can't get simpler than that.

● SUGAR IS NOT THE PROBLEM

When I tell people that sugar is not their problem, they often protest. They *know* that the cakes, pies, brownies, and cookies they've been eating contributed to their expanding waistlines. And they're right. These foods are a major contributor to America's growing weight problem, but it's not so much because of the sugar in them as it is the combination of sugar and starch.

Starch is tasteless. If you don't believe that, try eating a spoonful of flour. You can hardly taste anything. It just feels as if you have a bunch of paste in your mouth. Sugar, on the other hand, is sickeningly sweet. Try eating a spoonful of *that*; it's nauseating. However, if you mix the two—if you put sugar in baked goods, such as cookies, cakes, and pies—you give the flour some flavor and you hide much of the sweetness of the sugar. The sugar makes you consume more starch, and the starch makes you consume more sugar. You end up eating a lot more starch and sugar than you would normally have the desire to eat. And as good as it might taste, it all turns to sugar in your gut.

So cookies, cakes, and doughnuts are out if you're trying to reduce your glycemic load, but here's the good news. The glycemic loads of sweets that *do not contain starch* are not particularly high—much lower, in fact, than the glycemic loads of starches, such as bread, potatoes, and rice. The table below lists the glycemic loads of some popular foods. As you can see, the glycemic loads of dark chocolate, peanut M&M's, and even pure table sugar aren't too bad.

GLYCEMIC LOADS OF POPULAR FOODS	GLYCEMIC LOAD (PERCENTAGE OF 1 SLICE OF WHITE BREAD)
Life Saver, 1 piece	20
Sugar, 1 rounded teaspoon	28
Peanut M&M's, 1 snack-size bag	43
Dark chocolate, two 1" squares	44
Licorice, 1 twist	45
White chocolate, two 1" squares	49
Milk chocolate, two 1" squares	68
White bread, 1 slice	**100**
Doughnut, 1 medium-size	205
Cupcake, 2$^{1}/_{2}$" diameter	213
Brown rice, 1 cup	**222**
Baked potato, 1 potato	**246**

Notice that the glycemic loads of the candies are lower than those of the bread, potatoes, and rice. How could that be? It's not that they don't contain high concentrations of easily digestible sugar. It's because *the typical serving sizes are smaller.* Certainly, if you ate a pile of candy the size of a baked potato or a plateful of rice, you would raise your blood sugar as much as you would if you ate a baked potato or a plateful of rice. However, most of us don't need that much candy to satisfy the urge for something sweet. A handful will usually do.

Why don't we eat as large portions of candy as we do bread, potatoes, or rice? Because most of us have a limited tolerance for sweetness. Although starch is pure sugar, the molecules are bonded together, so you can't taste the sweetness—only about 2 percent of it breaks down to sugar in your mouth. However, you can taste *all* of the sugar in candy, so you need less of it to satisfy your sweet tooth. Indeed, despite skyrocketing

HIGH-FRUCTOSE CORN SYRUP: SUGAR BY **Another Name**

IN THE PAST 40 YEARS, as we have become more overweight and diabetic, we have been consuming less old-fashioned cane sugar and more high-fructose corn syrup (HFCS). Is there anything about this sweetener that could be contributing to these problems?

Actually, HFCS contains the same sugars that are in cane sugar: glucose and fructose. The only difference is that cane sugar is 50 percent fructose and HFCS is 55 percent fructose. There really isn't much difference, but even if there were, there's nothing unnatural about fructose. It's the main sugar in fruit. In fact, your body turns all sugar to fructose before metabolizing it.

The problem is mainly an economic one: High-fructose corn syrup is much cheaper than cane sugar. It slashes the cost of manufacturing sweets, which makes them much cheaper for consumers. This is especially true of soda. Now kids can afford to buy pop in 32-ounce Big Gulp containers instead of 7-ounce bottles, which were typical in the 1950s and '60s. Drinking so much soda in one sitting would have been inconceivable in the past.

Sodas are now the largest single source of calories for children and teenagers. They account for most of the increased sweetener consumption that has occurred in the past 40 years and are a major contributor to America's epidemic of childhood obesity.

obesity and diabetes rates, Americans aren't eating any more candy than they did 50 years ago. According to USDA statistics, average candy consumption hasn't changed since the 1960s.

Because diabetics have problems with high blood levels of glucose, which, of course, is a type of sugar, doctors used to think that the worst thing a diabetic could do was consume sugar—the kind we use to sweeten things. However, the glycemic load measurements cast sugar in a different light. The glycemic load of a teaspoon of sugar is only 28 percent of that of a slice of white bread. If you want to put a teaspoon of sugar in your coffee or tea or sprinkle it on some berries, it's not going to raise your daily glycemic load much at all.

In fact, if you're trying to reduce your glycemic load, sugar can actually help. It's natural to crave a hint of sweetness. We have tastebuds devoted specifically to detecting sugar. To prehistoric hunter-gatherers, the taste of sugar meant that a plant part was edible and a source of calories. It is not surprising that for many of us, a meal isn't complete without something sweet for dessert. The fact that many sweets have reasonably low glycemic loads is good news for those of us with a sweet tooth. A few bites of candy after a meal will have little effect on your blood sugar or on your body's demand for insulin, and can be quite satisfying. Indeed, it's a lot easier to pass up the potatoes and rice if you can look forward to something sweet for dessert.

And, honestly, did you really think you could live without sweets?

It's true that for some people, sugar has an addictive quality. It can trigger bingelike behavior. They intend to eat one piece of chocolate and end up consuming the whole box. If that's true for you, you should avoid sweets altogether. However, most of us can satisfy the urge for something sweet with just a few bites.

So it's okay to keep some candy around; just make sure it doesn't contain starch—no cookies, cakes, pie, or pastries. Use sweets to satisfy your sweet tooth, not to fill up on. If you're still hungry, have more meat and vegetables. Here are two rules of thumb for eating sweets: Eat them for dessert only, and don't eat more than you can hold in the cup of your hand.

Sugar Substitutes

CANE SUGAR, everybody's favorite sweetener, is pure sucrose, a double molecule of glucose and fructose. Enzymes in your small intestine split sucrose into its component sugars before it enters your bloodstream. Thus, when you consume cane sugar, you're actually consuming glucose and fructose.

To cut costs, food producers are using increasing amounts of high-fructose corn syrup in place of cane sugar. This sweetener contains the same sugars as cane sugar: glucose and fructose. The only difference is slightly more fructose—55 percent versus 50 percent.

Also popular are so-called natural sugars such as whole cane sugar (Sucanat), honey, and agave nectar. Although whole cane sugar and honey have interesting taste overtones, their composition is largely the same as sucrose: equal parts glucose and fructose. Their effect on blood sugar and insulin levels is no different from that of cane sugar. Agave nectar is higher in fructose, which makes it sweeter than cane sugar.

The sweeter a sweetener is, the less of it you need to sweeten things up. Consequently, using agave nectar as a sweetener should encourage you to consume less sugar.

Sugar-free sweeteners provide sweetness but with negligible calories. The four most popular ones are aspartame (Equal, NutraSweet), saccharin (Sweet'n Low), sucralose (Splenda, Altern), and stevia. Food producers also use sugar alcohols (sorbitol and maltitol) to sweeten their products. Although some scientists have expressed concern about the safety of artificial sweeteners, they have been extensively researched and to date have not been shown to be harmful. The FDA has deemed all of the above to be safe.

Artificial sweeteners have no effect on blood sugar. It should be noted, however, that, despite their widespread use in the past 40 years, they have not prevented our obesity and diabetes epidemics—consistent with the premise that starch, not sugar, is the main dietary culprit.

● SUGAR-SWEETENED BEVERAGES

Whereas a modest helping of candy shouldn't drive up your blood sugar enough to worry about, sugar-sweetened beverages are another matter. The glycemic loads of sodas, sports drinks, and even most fruit juices rank right up there with the starches.

In many ways, sugar-sweetened beverages behave like starches in your digestive system. Like starches, they release a lot of sugar into your bloodstream, and as with starches, you taste only a fraction of the sugar in beverages—but not because the sugar molecules are bound together as they are in starch. It's because your mouth handles liquids and solids differently. You don't chew beverages; you gulp them. Most of the sugar shoots over your tongue without coming in contact with your tastebuds. To make matters worse, we obscure the taste of sugar by cooling our beverages and adding sour things like lemon or lime, which neutralize the sweetness in them.

The worst offenders are sodas. A 12-ounce can of Coke contains the equivalent of 10 teaspoons of sugar, all of which rushes into your bloodstream within minutes of your drinking it. Harvard researchers reported in the *Journal of the American Medical Association* that adults who consume one or more sugar-sweetened beverages per day double their risk of developing diabetes within 4 years.

Of course, if you're concerned about your weight or you have diabetes, you already knew that you should avoid soda. However, fruit juices—even without added sugar—are almost as bad. Think about it: You don't have to add sugar to fruit juice to come up with a sugar-sweetened beverage. All the sugar in fruit is in the juice. When you take the juice from several pieces of fruit and put it all in one glass, you, in effect, create a sugar-sweetened beverage. You also leave behind the natural sugar blockers—the cellulose barriers, cell walls, and fiber.

Even if you include the whole fruit—for example, if you make a smoothie by pulverizing fruit in a blender—consuming fruit in liquid form increases its glycemic load. The reason is that you tend to consume more fruit when it's liquefied than you do when you eat it whole. In other words, the serving sizes are larger.

One reason sugar-sweetened beverages tend to make people fat is that, despite containing plenty of calories, they don't curb your hunger. In a study reported in the *International Journal of Obesity and Related Metabolic Disorders,* researchers at Purdue University had a group of subjects consume 450 calories a day in the form of jelly beans and another group the same amount of calories in sugar-sweetened beverages, then kept track of the number of calories they consumed for 4 weeks. The group that ate the jelly beans reduced the number of calories they ate by approximately the same number of calories that they consumed in the jelly beans. The group that drank the sugar-sweetened beverages did not reduce their food consumption at all. Sugar-containing beverages have the unique effect of adding to calories from other foods rather than replacing them.

In a way, the fact that sugar-sweetened beverages don't suppress appetite is good news. Usually, if you try to eliminate a particular food from your diet, you end up eating more of others. But just as consuming sugar-containing beverages doesn't reduce your appetite, eliminating them *doesn't increase your appetite.* It's a freebie—you can reduce calories without increasing hunger. People who drink sugar-containing beverages are often surprised at how easy it is to lose weight when they give them up. My medical assistant, Nadine Warner, tried to lose weight for years. When she found out how much sugar was in the two Frappuccinos she was drinking every day, she switched to coffee and cream, lost 20 pounds in 3 months, and has kept the weight off for 2 years.

● WHAT ABOUT ICE CREAM?

The glycemic load of a modest helping ($^1/_4$ cup) of full-fat ice cream is reasonable enough—30 to 40 percent of that of a slice of white bread. Remember, though, that ice cream is a sugar-sweetened liquid, albeit a frozen one. It behaves like a beverage in your mouth. You gulp it rather than chew it, so you don't taste as much of the sugar as you do in solid sweets. Also, the coldness blunts its taste. You might find yourself consuming more than a modest helping to satisfy your sweet tooth.

And don't bother with low-fat ice creams. They usually contain more sugar than the full-fat varieties do. Some brands have glycemic loads as high as 70. Now you can buy full-fat ice creams with no added sugar.

Although full-fat, unsweetened yogurts have glycemic loads as low as 10 percent of that of a slice of white bread, most commercial fruit-flavored yogurts have glycemic loads higher than 100 and should be avoided. It seems that most commercial flavored yogurts are sweetened to accommodate the tastes of kids. Here's a good trick: Use plain, full-fat, unsweetened yogurt; add fresh fruit; and sweeten to suit your taste. Put the sugar directly on the fruit. You'll probably find that you need only $^1/_2$ teaspoon or so of sugar, which has a glycemic load of 14, to bring out the flavor of the fruit.

● NONCULPRITS

Anyone who has succeeded in breaking a bad habit will tell you that you can take on only one habit at a time and succeed. This is especially true of diet. People tend to overestimate their ability to stop eating foods they're accustomed to. When they find that they're unable to avoid them, they often quit trying to change altogether. The less you have to change, the greater your chances of success. The key is to focus on eliminating as few foods as possible. Now that you've learned to identify the culprits, you need to recognize the "nonculprits"—foods the avoidance of which may serve only to reduce your satisfaction and lessen your chances of success.

JIM AND TAMMY HOBAR

JIM AND TAMMY HOBAR found themselves simultaneously approaching middle age and type 2 diabetes. Tammy knew that she was at risk by being overweight, and her blood test results indicated that she was "prediabetic." Jim, too, was struggling with weight and high blood pressure, and also has a strong familial history of diabetes.

In the past, Jim and Tammy had shed pounds on other weight loss plans but found themselves hungry a lot. However, with the Sugar Blockers Diet, Tammy reported: "I'm not as hungry as frequently. I was more successful than on the other diets because I wasn't starving, I was able to feel full longer, and so I didn't quit." Both were even able to keep up the program during a family vacation to Hawaii.

Sugar blocking paid off. Tammy lost an astonishing 9½ inches from her waist, chest, hip, thighs, and arms! Jim lost 6 inches. "People at work said I was looking like I lost weight in my face and neck," he said.

Sugar blocking did much more for this duo than help them shave some poundage. Their way of thinking, especially when it came to grocery shopping and eating out, completely changed. "We were definitely not eating well beforehand," said Tammy. "Overall, we are eating much better."

You've learned that reducing refined carbohydrates will help you lose weight and prevent or control diabetes. However, you've also been told that dietary fat makes you fat, the cholesterol in food gives you high blood cholesterol, salt raises your blood pressure, and trans fats (a by-product of

Jim, who does the grocery shopping for the household, found himself paying more attention to his task. "I've started reading labels more," he said. Tammy said her hubby no longer just brings home the bacon; he brings home fresh fruit and veggies!

Best of all, both have significantly reduced their high blood pressure. Tammy, whose doctor recently put her on blood pressure medication, is looking to come off it as a result of this program. "My hope is to stay off the medicine; that's the goal," she said.

They also log more hours at the gym than before. Tammy noted: "I was at the highest weight I've ever been at. I was achy . . . and now I don't have that anymore, no pain. Instead, I have a bicep muscle!" Jim reported, "My joints don't ache anymore, and my energy is better."

With blood pressure down, pain erased, and pounds and inches falling off left and right, it looks like nothing but good things on the horizon for the Hobars as they continue to eat the Sugar Blockers Diet way. "It's not that hard," said Jim. "You find what you like to eat and it's going to work."

JIM
Age: 45
Lost 8½ pounds
and 6"
in 6 weeks

●

TAMMY
Age: 42
Lost 8 pounds
and 9½"
in 6 weeks

commercially processed oils) damage your arteries. The truth is that if you cut out all of the foods you hear bad things about, you'd hardly have anything left to eat.

So let's look at these presumed culprits one at a time.

Salt. The fact is that no one has proved that you can prevent high blood pressure or cardiovascular disease by avoiding salt. It's debatable that dietary salt has anything to do with high blood pressure. In a recent European study reported in the *Journal of the American Medical Association,* among more than 3,600 participants tracked for 8 years, researchers found that reduced salt intake did not prevent high blood pressure and actually *increased* the risk of cardiovascular disease.

One thing is not debatable: The best thing you can do to avoid high blood pressure and heart disease is to have a normal body weight—and the best way to do that, as you've learned, is to avoid refined carbs.

Trans fats. In the 1960s, companies started promoting foods made with unsaturated fats, such as vegetable oil, as healthy alternatives to saturated fats, the kind in suet and lard. However, these products didn't keep as well as those made with saturated fats. Unsaturated fat becomes rancid after a few days at room temperature. To solve this problem, manufacturers developed a process called partial hydrogenation, which extends the shelf life of foods made with unsaturated fat.

Scientists recently discovered a problem with partially hydrogenated fats. The hydrogenation process produces an unnatural kind of fat called trans fat, which not only raises bad cholesterol but also lowers good cholesterol. Several cities have now banned products that contain excessive amounts of trans fat.

The good news is that if you avoid refined carbohydrates, you don't have to worry about trans fat. Most of the partially hydrogenated fats in our diet are consumed with starches. If you avoid packaged flour products, such as cookies, crackers, and chips, you avoid the commercial oils used to prepare them. If you cut out bread and potatoes, you eliminate the margarine you used to eat with them. You'll have hardly any trans fat in your diet at all.

Fat and cholesterol. There was a time when low-carb diets were thought to be unhealthy because they encouraged people to eat more fat and cholesterol. If you eliminate carbs, you have to eat something to replace them, so you tend to eat more eggs, meat, and dairy products. However, the notion that cholesterol-containing foods are unhealthy has been thoroughly disproved. Study after study has shown that low-carbohydrate, unrestricted-fat-and-cholesterol diets actually improve the balance between good and bad cholesterol, which reduces the risk of heart disease.

How did the notion that eggs, meat, and dairy products are bad for us get so firmly entrenched in the minds of Americans?

In the 1950s, researchers discovered that patients who had heart attacks often had high levels of cholesterol in their blood. Taking literally the old saw "You are what you eat," some scientists assumed, *without proof,* that high blood cholesterol came from eating too many cholesterol-containing foods. For their part, doctors never noticed any tendency for eggs, dairy products, and red meat to cause heart problems. Most physicians at the time did not advise their patients to avoid cholesterol.

Then the US government got involved. In the 1960s, a congressional committee charged with combating malnutrition concluded that lack of food was no longer a problem in the United States. Faced with having to disband for want of a mission, the committee decided to investigate the issue of *over*nutrition. Some congressmen—none of whom was trained in medicine—met with a few researchers who discussed the premise that cholesterol-containing foods cause heart disease. The logic of "You are what you eat" sounded reasonable to them. They passed the idea on to the other committee members, who used it as a reason for the committee's continued existence. For the first time in its history, the US government took upon itself the task of getting people to reduce their consumption of an entire category of food.

The idea of reducing dietary cholesterol appealed to the experts at the time for other reasons. Cholesterol comes from animal products, which also contain fat. They figured that if high blood cholesterol comes from eating cholesterol-containing food, maybe fatness comes from eating fat-containing foods. If you avoid animal products, perhaps you could lose weight as well as reduce your cholesterol level. Also, reducing cholesterol consumption is kinder to animals and easier on people's pocketbooks. Eggs, meat, and dairy products are more expensive than starchy staples like bread, potatoes, and rice. If folks didn't eat so many animal products, they could prevent heart disease, slim down, save money, be nicer to animals, and save the planet all at the same time.

The problem was, the theory was wrong.

Make no mistake: High levels of cholesterol in your blood—or, more precisely, imbalances between good and bad cholesterol—*can* clog up your arteries and cause heart disease. However, high blood cholesterol decidedly does *not* come from eating cholesterol-containing foods, nor does avoiding dietary cholesterol prevent high blood cholesterol. What scientists then didn't realize is that your body makes most of its own cholesterol. If you eat less, it just makes more, and vice versa. Actually, the cholesterol in food is difficult to digest. Most of it passes right through your intestinal tract and out in your stool.

● DR. ATKINS MEETS MR. BANTING

In 1864, an overweight British undertaker named William Banting, having failed to lose weight after trying several different schemes, consulted a prominent London physician who recommended that he concentrate on eliminating starch and sugar from his diet. When this proved successful, Banting published a pamphlet about the diet, which was widely read in Europe and America. For almost a century, people used his name as a verb, saying they were "banting" when they were avoiding carbohydrates.

Cutting carbs continued to be the most popular way to lose weight until the 1970s, when doctors, impressed with the government's warnings about the dangers of cholesterol, started recommending the opposite approach: cutting out fat and cholesterol, and eating *more* carbohydrates. Although it wasn't apparent until decades later, this was when America's obesity and diabetes epidemics began.

Because diabetes raises the risk of blood vessel disease, diabetes experts became convinced that people with diabetes would benefit by reducing dietary cholesterol. This actually encouraged diabetes patients to eat *more* starch, which, of course, made their diabetes more difficult to control. However, the pharmaceutical industry came up with what looked like a solution: pills that spurred people's beta cells to make more insulin. The experts at the time figured that folks with type 2 diabetes could use pills to keep their blood sugar down.

This high-carb, low-fat, pill-popping approach was standard treatment until the early 1990s, when a New York City cardiologist named Robert Atkins blew out of the water the notion that people should avoid cholesterol. Essentially, he rediscovered banting. For years Atkins had observed that his patients could eat all of the eggs, meat, and dairy products they wanted and still lose weight as long as they avoided carbohydrates. He crafted a low-carbohydrate diet, with no restrictions on fat and cholesterol, that he published in 1992 in a book called *Dr. Atkins' New Diet Revolution.* The book was wildly popular.

At first Dr. Atkins was criticized by the medical establishment, which thought his diet would raise blood cholesterol levels and cause heart problems. However, Dr. Atkins was an experienced heart specialist. He knew from years of treating patients that reducing carbohydrates and increasing dietary fat and cholesterol doesn't raise levels of bad, or LDL, cholesterol. In fact, it raises levels of good, or HDL, cholesterol, which protects against blood vessel disease. Reducing carbohydrates also lowers triglyceride levels as well as blood sugar and insulin levels. Patients of his who cut carbs lost weight and seemed healthier.

In the late 1990s, with pressure from the public, researchers put the Atkins diet to the test. They conducted studies comparing his diet with the low-fat diets that other doctors were recommending. They found that Dr. Atkins was right. Subjects who followed a low-carbohydrate diet, without restricting fat and cholesterol and *without trying to reduce calories*, lost more weight than did those on low-fat diets *who tried to cut calories*. Cholesterol levels didn't increase. In fact, the balance between good and bad cholesterol—the most accurate predictor of heart disease—actually improved. Sadly, Dr. Atkins died in an accident a month before the nation's most reputable medical journal, the *New England Journal of Medicine,* published the results of those studies in 2003.

Actually, by 2000 it had already become apparent to most heart specialists that the low-cholesterol diets that they had been recommending since the 1970s didn't prevent heart disease. In fact, these diets didn't even lower cholesterol levels much. Every time they were put to the test, they had minimal effect on cholesterol levels and no discernible effect on heart disease. Nevertheless, the message to avoid cholesterol persisted in the minds of Americans.

To answer, once and for all, the question of whether or not low-cholesterol diets were beneficial, the National Institutes of Health commissioned a massive study called the Women's Health Initiative. It was the largest, most methodically conducted, and most expensive dietary trial ever done.

Researchers gave 19,000 women 18 sessions of low-fat, low-cholesterol dietary training in the first year of the study and a refresher session every 3 months until the end of the study. They compared this group with a similar-size group of women who did not receive the training. After 8 years, surveys showed that the women who received the training indeed reduced their fat and cholesterol consumption. The result? Eating less fat and cholesterol did virtually nothing. The average blood cholesterol level in the women who followed the low-fat, low-cholesterol diet fell less than 2 percent. In 8 years they lost only 2 pounds, and there was no decrease whatsoever in heart or blood vessel disease.

Again, make no mistake: *High blood cholesterol causes heart disease.* It's just that low-fat, low-cholesterol diets do not reduce blood cholesterol levels enough to make a difference. In Chapter 14 you'll learn that there are better ways to improve your cholesterol balance.

As a result of new insights into the benefits of low-carbohydrate diets and the lack of any benefits of low-fat, low-cholesterol diets, many doctors have returned to the time-honored approach of telling patients trying to lose weight or manage diabetes not to worry about fat and cholesterol but to concentrate on eliminating carbohydrates. They're rediscovering what Banting knew some 150 years ago: The best way to lose weight and treat diabetes is to reduce carbohydrates.

The Problem with Low-Carb Diets (and It's Not Cholesterol)

While there's little doubt that cutting carbs is an effective way to lose weight and prevent or treat diabetes, there's a problem with strict low-carbohydrate regimens like the Atkins diet: Most people simply can't stay on them for long. You might think that a diet that lets you eat as much rich food—eggs, butter, cheese, steak—as you want would be easy to follow, and, in fact, most people have little trouble staying on it at first. However, after a week or two, you start craving the missing foods—fruits, vegetables, milk products, starches, and sweets. Eventually the cravings become irresistible, and you go back to your old ways.

There's a reason for food cravings. It's Mother Nature's way of making sure you get the right balance of nutrients in your diet. You can't live on calories alone. You need vitamins, minerals, protein, and certain kinds of fats in your diet to stay healthy. Most of the foods we eat contain nutrients that are necessary for good health. When your diet falls short of providing some vital nutrient, your body lets you know by causing you to crave foods that contain it.

Fruits and vegetables are full of vitamins, antioxidants, minerals, and fiber that are essential to good health. Meat and dairy products are rich sources of protein and fats that you can't live without. There's even a biological reason for craving sugar: To prehistoric humans, sweetness meant that a plant part was safe to eat and a good source of calories. It's not surprising that removing fruits, vegetables, dairy products, and sweets from your diet triggers cravings.

Of course, food cravings aren't confined to strict low-carbohydrate diets. Low-*fat* diets are even worse. In addition to eliminating satisfying rich foods and your main sources of protein, essential fats, and many vitamins, you consciously have to cut calories. Besides craving the missing foods, you get just plain hungry.

So what can you do? You know that carbohydrates raise your blood sugar, cause weight gain, throw your cholesterol out of balance, increase your blood pressure, burn out your insulin-making cells, and put you at risk for a host of other medical problems. But when you try to cut out carbohydrates, you're hit by irresistible food cravings.

It seems like a dilemma until you recall that it's not just the number of carbohydrates you eat that determines your body's demands for insulin;

it's how quickly they break down to sugar and enter your bloodstream. You don't have to avoid all carbs, just the ones that cause your blood sugar and insulin levels to spike after you eat them. You can continue eating many carbohydrates; benefit from the vitamins, minerals, and fiber they provide; and even enjoy sweets without overloading your system with glucose and insulin, if you just avoid those high–glycemic load culprits: the starches and sugar-containing beverages.

● AN EATING STYLE YOU CAN LIVE WITH

Thirty years of counseling people about their eating habits have taught me that, if there's one dietary change people are capable of making, it's reducing the amount of starch they eat. Remember, starch is basically tasteless. When you remove it from your diet and replace it with other foods, you actually increase the flavor in your diet. Starch contains no essential vitamins or minerals, so when you stop eating it, you experience no natural food cravings. You can eat tastier foods—and more of them—while reducing your glycemic load. When you get rid of after-meal blood sugar spikes, you eliminate the main cause of weight gain: excessive insulin secretion. Research studies have proved over and over that when you cut out starch, *even if you don't try to reduce calories,* you usually end up losing more weight than if you go on a low-fat diet and try to cut calories.

You don't need to say good-bye to all of your favorite foods. You don't even need to worry about sugar—as long you use a little restraint. Assuming that you're not foolish enough to keep drinking sugar-containing beverages, that leaves just one kind of food you need to limit: starches. Can a diet get any easier than that?

Well, maybe just a little. Wouldn't it be nice if you could eat the occasional serving of pasta, slice of bread, or piece of cake without wreaking havoc on your blood sugar? This is where sugar blockers come in.

6

NATURE'S MOST ABUNDANT SUGAR BLOCKER

THE FACT that you can reduce your body's needs for insulin to a fraction of what they usually are by cutting out starches is great news. Nevertheless, a lot of us still find it difficult to eliminate refined carbohydrates altogether. We develop a taste for starch when we are very young. Our mothers, anxious to wean us from milk, start us on refined carbs early in life because starch is so easy to digest. Indeed, recent studies show that the earlier in life kids start eating it, the greater their chances of becoming obese later. We use bread, potatoes, rice, and pasta as "filler foods," cheap sources of calories. Dietary custom born of economic necessity dictates that some kind of refined carbohydrates be included with virtually every meal we eat. Sometimes it's downright awkward to avoid these foods.

So how can you lower your blood sugar, reduce your body's needs for insulin, and lose weight without completely eliminating refined carbohydrates? You can reduce the effects of such foods on your blood sugar and insulin requirements by taking advantage of natural substances in foods that slow carbohydrate digestion and blunt after-meal glucose spikes.

You see, starches have a very peculiar digestive pattern. We are endowed with approximately 22 feet of small intestine. Other foods require most of that length in order to be broken down and absorbed. Nutrients slowly trickle into the bloodstream over the course of several hours. But refined carbohydrates don't travel 2 feet before they rush into your bloodstream. Our bodies digest starches at warp speed. The good news is that there are ways you can slow down that process. Many natural foods rein in runaway digestion and reduce starch's effects on your blood sugar and insulin requirements. Nature's most abundant sugar blocker is what food scientists call soluble fiber.

● WHAT IS FIBER?

Only a tiny fraction of the vegetation on Earth is digestible. The glucose molecules in most plants are linked by strong bonds called beta bonds, which the digestive systems of most animals cannot break. (This contrasts with the weak alpha bonds that hold together the glucose molecules in starch.) Glucose molecules held together by those strong beta bonds pass through your intestinal tract as indigestible material—that is, fiber.

Fiber provides the structure material of plants. By encasing the digestible parts of fruits and vegetables in peels, husks, stalks, and cell walls, and by soaking up glucose like a sponge, fiber creates physical barriers to digestion. Your digestive system can break down some of these barriers and absorb the sugar and starch they protect, but that takes time. Glucose slowly seeps into your bloodstream over several hours.

Insoluble Fiber

Nutritionists recognize two kinds of fiber: insoluble and soluble. Insoluble fiber passes through your digestive tract chemically unchanged. It forms the husks and peels of fruits and vegetables—parts we often don't eat. That's unfortunate, because insoluble fiber is vital for colon health. It prevents constipation and promotes regularity. Lack of insoluble fiber triggers irritable bowel syndrome, which is a common cause of gassiness, bloating, and abdominal discomfort, and causes diverticulosis—pouches in the colon that can bleed or become infected.

For millions of years, prehistoric humans ate what we would consider huge amounts of insoluble fiber in such things as roots, bark, grasses, and unripe fruits and vegetables. The vegetation they ate was so difficult to digest, it provided barely enough calories to prevent starvation. Consequently, our digestive systems evolved to handle large amounts of insoluble fiber. However, the carbohydrates we eat now are so refined that they're practically devoid of this kind of fiber. Indeed, lack of insoluble fiber is the only unquestioned, widespread dietary deficiency in industrialized countries. Whereas the optimal amount for good health is probably upwards of 20 grams per day, most Americans eat less than a few grams per day.

The best source of insoluble fiber in the American diet is wheat "bran"—wheat husks without the starch. For years, millers considered bran a worthless by-product of the flour-making process. They sold it by the barrel to farmers as cheap cattle feed. However, once people figured out how helpful bran was for colon health, companies began making it into breakfast cereal. Now it's advertised on television and sold at prices many times higher than cattle feed.

One-half cup of bran cereal provides 12 grams of insoluble fiber. You can also get some insoluble fiber from nuts, seeds, and the peels and stalks of some fruits and vegetables.

Soluble Fiber

Soluble fiber, unlike the insoluble kind, is abundant in the parts of fruits and vegetables that we do eat. Although soluble fiber is not as effective as insoluble fiber for preventing constipation and relieving irritable bowel syndrome, it is a much more effective sugar blocker. It slows the absorption not only of glucose in the foods that contain it but also of *the glucose released by other foods*. Here's how it works.

As soluble fiber passes through your intestinal tract, it takes up fluid, swells, and gradually changes from solid to gel. As it swells, it soaks up fluid like a sponge, trapping starch and sugar in the niches between its molecules. "Soluble" means dissolvable—and indeed, soluble fiber eventually dissolves, and the glucose it soaks up gets washed out and absorbed into your bloodstream. However, that takes time. The glucose it absorbs seeps into your bloodstream slowly, so your body needs less insulin to handle it. Soluble fiber has been found to produce significant reductions in blood sugar in 33 of 50 studies testing it. In clinical intervention trials ranging from 2 to 17 weeks, the consumption of fiber was shown to decrease insulin requirements in people with type 2 diabetes.

In addition to fiber, many fruits and vegetables contain substances that evolved specifically to deactivate digestive enzymes. Their purpose in nature is to protect plants from being consumed by insects and bacteria, which, like us, have enzymes for digesting starch and sugar.

Soluble fiber also exerts what scientists call the "second-meal effect"—it reduces blood sugar not only after the meal with which it is consumed but also after the next meal of the day. Researchers at the University of Virginia gave soluble fiber to subjects with their breakfast and measured blood sugar levels before and after both breakfast and lunch. They compared their results with measurements in subjects who received no added fiber. The soluble fiber both lowered glucose after the breakfast meal and reduced the after-lunch glucose surge by 31 percent, compared with the after-lunch surge of the subjects who were not given added fiber.

Some scientists believe that soluble fiber helps protect against heart disease. Besides reducing blood sugar and insulin levels, it has a modest blood cholesterol–lowering effect. It does this by soaking up cholesterol in the intestinal tract.

"Wait a minute," you're thinking. "Didn't he say that cholesterol in food doesn't matter?" That's right, most of the cholesterol in your blood does *not* come from cholesterol in food—your body makes it. However, soluble fiber binds not just to cholesterol in food but also to cholesterol produced by your body. Your liver secretes bile into your intestine, and bile contains a form of cholesterol called bile acid, which is normally absorbed back into your bloodstream. Soluble fiber traps this kind of cholesterol and carries it out in the stool. Phytosterols, a type of vegetable fat abundant in oily vegetables such as nuts and olives, have a similar effect. In a study reported in the *Journal of the American Medical Association,* University of Toronto researchers were able to reduce cholesterol levels as much as some statins can, by giving subjects large amounts of soluble fiber along with phytosterol supplements.

Although there are plenty of good sources of soluble fiber in the fruits and vegetables we eat, we still tend to eat less of it than we should. Food scientists recommend that we consume 25 grams per day, but most Americans consume fewer than 5 grams.

● BALANCING FIBER CONTENT VERSUS SUGAR CONTENT

You may have heard that whole grain products are high in fiber. However, the starch in grains quickly turns to sugar and overwhelms any sugar-blocking effect the fiber might have. Of course, all fruits and vegetables contain sugar; that's what makes them carbohydrates. Nevertheless, most contain proportionately more soluble fiber than sugar, so they don't raise blood sugar as much as grain products and other refined carbohydrates do.

You can tell which fruits and vegetables have the best balance of fiber to sugar by looking at their glycemic loads. All of the carbohydrates that have been associated with increased risk of obesity or diabetes have glycemic loads greater than 100. On the other hand, fruits and vegetables with glycemic loads less than 100 have been associated with reduced risk. Thus, you should avoid fruits or vegetables with glycemic loads higher than 100, even though they contain soluble fiber. Fruits and vegetables whose glycemic loads are between 50 and 100 are themselves acceptable to eat, but they release enough glucose to nullify their usefulness as sugar blockers. The best fruit and vegetable sugar blockers are those with glycemic loads less than 50. Throughout this chapter you'll find tables that show the fiber content of various foods as well as their glycemic loads so that you can choose the best sources of fiber.

It takes about 10 grams of fiber to reduce the after-meal blood sugar surge from a serving of starch by approximately 25 percent. As you will see, no single, typical serving of fruits or vegetables comes close to providing the 10 grams needed to lower your blood sugar by 25 percent; you would need to include several portions.

A good way to ensure that you get enough soluble fiber to do the job is to have a salad with your meal—preferably before you eat starch. Salads allow you to combine enough sugar blockers to have a beneficial effect. For example, a salad containing 2 cups of romaine (2 grams of fiber), a cup of chopped tomatoes (2 grams), and a cup of red bell peppers (3 grams) provides 7 grams of fiber. Add that, say, to a cup of broccoli (4.5 grams) with your meal and you have 11.5 grams of fiber.

Soluble fiber blocks sugar best when consumed before, rather than after, you eat starch. For instance, if your meal includes a salad, steak, potatoes, and green beans, eat the salad and at least some of the green beans before eating the potatoes.

● FRUITS

One difference between fruits and vegetables is that nature intended fruits to be eaten by birds and beasts. That's how they spread their seeds. Animals are enticed by the sugar in fruit. However, the generous sugar content of some fruits counteracts some of their usefulness as sugar blockers. Thanks to the second-meal effect, they might reduce glucose levels

Fiber Contents and Glycemic Loads of Fruits

FOOD	SERVING SIZE	FIBER (GRAMS)	ESTIMATED GLYCEMIC LOAD	EFFECT ON BLOOD SUGAR
Apricot	3 apricots	2.4	24	Sugar blocker
Avocado	1/2 avocado	3.5	20	Sugar blocker
Banana (all brown)	1 banana	2.8	105	High glycemic
Banana (all green)	1 banana	2.8	65	Acceptable
Banana (half green)	1 banana	2.8	85	Acceptable
Blackberries	1 cup	7.6	Less than 15	Sugar blocker
Blueberries	1 cup	3.9	40	Acceptable
Cantaloupe	1/4 cantaloupe	1.2	52	Acceptable
Cherries (pitted)	10 cherries	1.6	43	Acceptable
Dates	5 dates	3.2	298	High glycemic
Figs	5 figs	18	151	High glycemic
Grapefruit	1/2 grapefruit	1.4	32	Sugar blocker
Grapes	1/2 cup	0.8	47	Acceptable
Honeydew melon	1/4 melon	2	75	Acceptable
Kiwifruit	1 kiwifruit	2.6	43	Acceptable
Mango (cubed)	1/2 cup	1.5	67	Acceptable
Nectarines	1 nectarine	2.2	48	Acceptable
Orange	1 orange	3.1	43	Acceptable
Papaya (cubed)	1 cup	2.5	30	Sugar blocker
Peach	1 peach	2	47	Acceptable
Pear	1 pear	4	57	Acceptable
Pineapple (diced)	1 cup	1.9	52	Acceptable
Plantains (cooked)	1 cup	3.5	200	High glycemic
Plums (pitted)	2 plums	2	47	Acceptable
Prunes (dried, pitted)	5 prunes	3	65	Acceptable
Raspberries	1 cup	8.4	Less than 15	Sugar blocker
Strawberries	1 cup	3.8	Less than 15	Sugar blocker
Tangerine	1 tangerine	1.9	65	Acceptable
Watermelon (diced)	1 cup	0.8	30	Sugar blocker

after the *next* meal, but the sugar they release neutralizes the benefits for the *first* meal.

As fruit ripens, fiber barriers soften and the sugar content rises. Berries, peaches, and apricots have low glycemic loads even when fully ripe. Pears should be eaten while still crisp. Tart-tasting apples, such as Golden Delicious, make good sugar blockers, but the sweeter varieties, such as Fuji and Honeycrisp, contain enough sugar to counteract their usefulness as sugar blockers. Dried fruits have higher glycemic loads than fresh fruit simply because they're smaller, so you tend to eat more of them.

● VEGETABLES

As a rule, vegetables make better sugar blockers than fruits do. They have higher fiber contents and lower glycemic loads. Soluble fiber is, well, soluble, so it soaks up water. Boiling vegetables until they're limp and soggy saturates the soluble fiber in them, making them less effective as sugar blockers. Also, the more crisp that vegetables are when you eat them, the chunkier they will be when they reach your stomach. As we learned in Chapter 4, the larger the food particles, the longer it takes to digest them. Carrots, broccoli, cauliflower, green beans, and asparagus all work best when they're cooked just enough for you to be able to puncture their surface with a fork. The rawer they are, the more effective they are as sugar blockers. For example, Swedish researchers fed a group of subjects raw carrots with a starch-containing meal, and compared their after-meal blood sugar levels with those of a group that was fed cooked carrots. The subjects who ate the raw carrots with their meal not only had lower after-meal blood sugar and insulin levels; they also had significantly higher "satiety ratings," which measure how satisfied they felt.

In addition to their sugar-blocking effects, vegetables can often serve as delicious and satisfying starch substitutes. Said tester Jane Wilchak, "Roasted veggies and roasted cauliflowers—that became my new starch."

Fiber Contents and Glycemic Loads of Vegetables

FOOD	SERVING SIZE	FIBER (GRAMS)	ESTIMATED GLYCEMIC LOAD	EFFECT ON BLOOD SUGAR
Alfalfa sprouts	1 cup	0.8	Less than 15	Sugar blocker
Artichoke (cooked)	1 cup	9.1	Less than 15	Sugar blocker
Asparagus	1 cup	2.9	Less than 15	Sugar blocker
Bean sprouts	1 cup	1.9	Less than 15	Sugar blocker
Beets	½ cup	1.7	50	Acceptable
Broccoli	1 cup	4.5	Less than 15	Sugar blocker
Brussels sprouts	1 cup	4.1	40	Sugar blocker
Cabbage (cooked)	1 cup	3.5	Less than 15	Sugar blocker
Carrot (cooked)	1 cup	5.1	Less than 15	Sugar blocker
Carrot (raw)	One 7½" carrot	2.2	Less than 15	Sugar blocker
Cauliflower	1 cup	3.3	Less than 15	Sugar blocker
Celery (diced)	1 cup	2	Less than 15	Sugar blocker
Collard greens	1 cup	5.3	Less than 15	Sugar blocker
Cucumber (peeled)	1 cup	0.8	Less than 15	Sugar blocker
Cucumber pickle	1 large	1.6	Less than 15	Sugar blocker
Dandelion greens	1 cup	3	Less than 15	Sugar blocker
Eggplant	1 cup	2.5	Less than 15	Sugar blocker
Jerusalem artichoke	1 cup	2.4	150	High glycemic
Lettuce, butterhead	2 cups	1.1	Less than 15	Sugar blocker
Lettuce, iceberg	2 cups	1.6	Less than 15	Sugar blocker
Lettuce, looseleaf	2 cups	2.2	Less than 15	Sugar blocker
Lettuce, romaine	2 cups	2	Less than 15	Sugar blocker
Mushrooms (cooked)	1 cup	3.4	Less than 15	Sugar blocker
Mushrooms (raw)	1 cup	0.8	Less than 15	Sugar blocker
Mustard greens (cooked)	1 cup	2.8	Less than 15	Sugar blocker
Okra (cooked)	1 cup	4	Less than 15	Sugar blocker
Onions (cooked)	1 cup	2.9	Less than 15	Sugar blocker

FOOD	SERVING SIZE	FIBER (GRAMS)	ESTIMATED GLYCEMIC LOAD	EFFECT ON BLOOD SUGAR
Onions (raw)	½ cup	1.5	Less than 15	Sugar blocker
Parsnips (cooked)	½ cup	3.1	50	Acceptable
Peppers (green)	1 cup	2.7	Less than 15	Sugar blocker
Peppers (red)	1 cup	3	Less than 15	Sugar blocker
Potato (baked)	1 medium	4.8	264	High glycemic
Potato (flesh only)	1 medium	2.3	179	High glycemic
Potato skin (baked)	1 skin	2.5	85	Acceptable
Pumpkin (diced, cooked)	1 cup	2.7	180	High glycemic
Rutabaga	1 cup	3.1	70	Acceptable
Sauerkraut	1 cup	5.9	Less than 15	Sugar blocker
Scallions	1 cup	2.6	Less than 15	Sugar blocker
Spinach (cooked)	1 cup	4.3	Less than 15	Sugar blocker
Spinach (raw)	2 cups	1.6	Less than 15	Sugar blocker
Squash	1 cup	2.5	80	Acceptable
String beans	1 cup	4	Less than 15	Sugar blocker
Sweet potato	1 potato	4.4	170	High glycemic
Tomatoes (chopped)	1 cup	2	Less than 15	Sugar blocker
Turnip	1 cup	3.1	20	Sugar blocker
Turnip greens (cooked)	1 cup	5	Less than 15	Sugar blocker
Water chestnuts	½ cup	1.8	Less than 15	Sugar blocker

● BEANS

Beans and other legumes are packed with soluble fiber, but they also contain starch. A big serving can have a beneficial *second*-meal effect, but sometimes beans can release enough glucose to give you a sugar shock immediately after the first meal. Much depends on how you prepare them.

Fiber Contents and Glycemic Loads of Beans and Legumes

FOOD	SERVING SIZE	FIBER (GRAMS)	ESTIMATED GLYCEMIC LOAD	EFFECT ON BLOOD SUGAR
Beans, navy	½ cup	5.8	40	Sugar blocker
Beans, pinto	½ cup	7.4	45	Sugar blocker
Black-eyed peas	½ cup	6.6	74	Sugar blocker
Chickpeas	½ cup	6.2	45	Sugar blocker
Lentils	½ cup	7.8	30	Sugar blocker
Peas	½ cup	2.3	32	Sugar blocker
Soybeans	1 cup	7.6	Less than 15	Sugar blocker

If you start with uncooked beans and serve them slightly crisp, a ½ cup or so won't raise blood sugar much and can reduce the blood sugar–raising effects of other foods consumed during the first and second meals. It doesn't take a lot of beans for you to get a good dose of fiber; just a ½ cup can provide as much as 7.8 grams of fiber. And as you can see from the table above, if you stick to a ½-cup serving, you're in no danger of raising your glycemic load too high. However, if you cook them until they're mushy or let them sit overnight and then reheat them, they'll become starchier and will likely raise your blood sugar.

● NUTS AND SEEDS

Nuts not only are rich sources of fiber but also have other sugar-blocking qualities that will be discussed in the next chapter. In addition, they reduce levels of bad cholesterol and raise levels of good cholesterol. If you have the urge for a dry, crunchy snack, instead of going for the chips and crackers, which are pure starch, have some nuts instead. They're tasty and satisfying, and have negligible glycemic loads. You can eat them freely.

Unlike the seeds of wheat, rice, and corn, some other seeds have little starch and enough fiber to make good sugar blockers. Two sources of fiber with proven sugar-blocking qualities are chia seeds and flaxseeds.

Chia Seeds: Sugar-Absorbing Spheres

There's no food quite like chia seeds (*Salvia hispanica*). They're one of the tastiest ways to supplement your diet with fiber.

Imagine a balloon filling with water, and you'll have an idea how chia seeds work in your digestive tract. They look like grains of sand, but each particle is actually a round capsule filled with compact soluble fiber. As the seeds travel through your intestinal tract, they soak up fluid and expand to several times their original volume. The soluble fiber in them swells and absorbs glucose. Amazingly, the capsules remain intact, stretching like rubber water balloons, which keeps them in a spherical shape.

You can even watch them do this. Put a tablespoon of chia seeds in the bottom of a glass, and slowly add water. You can see the seeds swell up to several times their original size while maintaining their spherical shapes. (If you've ever owned a Chia Pet, you'll remember seeing this trick!)

Fiber Contents and Glycemic Loads of Nuts and Seeds

FOOD	SERVING SIZE	FIBER (GRAMS)	ESTIMATED GLYCEMIC LOAD	EFFECT ON BLOOD SUGAR
Almonds	24 nuts	3.2	Less than 15	Sugar blocker
Cashews	18 nuts	0.6	28	Sugar blocker
Chia seeds	1 Tbsp	5.5	Less than 15	Sugar blocker
Hazelnuts	20 nuts	2.7	Less than 15	Sugar blocker
Peanuts	28 nuts	2.3	Less than 15	Sugar blocker
Sunflower seeds	1/4 cup	2.9	Less than 15	Sugar blocker
Walnuts	14 halves	1.9	Less than 15	Sugar blocker

The speed with which soluble fiber dissolves depends on, among other things, its surface area. As it turns out, spheres have less surface area relative to their volume than do other shapes. Thus, the spherical configuration of the chia fiber globules keeps them from being dissolved as quickly as they otherwise would, and that slows the release of the glucose they soak up. University of Toronto researchers reported in the *Journal of the Federation of American Societies for Experimental Biology* that 1^1/$_2$ tablespoons of chia seeds reduces the blood sugar–raising effect of eating two slices of white bread by 33 percent.

Even before chia's beneficial effects on blood sugar were discovered, the seeds were known for their ability to improve bowel function. In addition to being an excellent source of soluble fiber, they contain plenty of the insoluble kind, which is essential for good colon health. Chia is unique in that it imparts a slippery consistency to stools, which further aids bowel function.

Chia seeds have a pleasant flavor, like tiny nuts. They're considered a delicacy in Latin America. You can add them to practically anything. They go especially well with dishes you might put nuts in—salads, vegetables, and even ice cream. One tester, Cindy Swan, carried chia seeds with her in her purse so that she could sprinkle them on restaurant salads.

Flaxseeds

Flaxseeds contain high concentrations of soluble fiber, insoluble fiber, and essential fatty acids. Like chia seeds, flaxseeds soak up glucose in your digestive tract, which slows its absorption. University of Toronto researchers reported in the *British Journal of Nutrition* that 3 rounded tablespoons with a meal reduces after-meal blood sugar surges by 25 to 30 percent. And as in chia seeds, the fiber in flaxseed improves bowel function.

Flaxseeds have a pleasant, nutty flavor. You can add them to anything you would sprinkle nuts in, including salads, fruit, and yogurt.

● FIBER-BOOSTING SUPPLEMENTS

Plant parts that contain particularly generous amounts of fiber are some-times used as dietary supplements. These include psyllium, oat bran, guar, pectin, and powdered seaweed, all of which have been shown to reduce after-meal blood sugar levels. You can buy these supplements in capsules or powder form at pharmacies or grocery stores.

As fiber soaks up fluid in your digestive tract, it softens and adds bulk to your stool. Fiber supplements are most often used to prevent constipa-tion and relieve irritable bowel syndrome, a common cause of abdominal discomfort and irregularity. However, like the natural fiber in fruits and vegetables, soluble fiber supplements can also reduce after-meal blood sugar and insulin demands. If you're already taking a fiber supplement—not a bad idea, considering that the typical American diet is markedly deficient in fiber—you can also put it to work as a sugar blocker.

To help slow carbohydrate absorption, you should take a fiber supplement shortly before eating. For example, if your evening meal is when you are most likely to eat starch, you should take it just before or during your meal.

Fiber Contents and Glycemic Loads of Fiber Supplements

SUPPLEMENT	SERVING SIZE	FIBER (GRAMS)	ESTIMATED GLYCEMIC LOAD	EFFECT ON BLOOD SUGAR
Guar gum	1 tsp	3	Less than 15	Sugar blocker
Metamucil	1 tsp	3	Less than 15	Sugar blocker
Oat bran (raw)	¼ cup	3.7	Less than 15	Sugar blocker
Psyllium husks	1 Tbsp	4.5	Less than 15	Sugar blocker

● MUSICAL FRUIT

As you start eating more fruits and vegetables, you might experience some gassiness, which usually subsides in a week or two. Instead of being absorbed in the first foot or two of the small intestine, as starchy foods are, the soluble fiber in fruits and vegetables travels the entire length of your intestine and arrives in your colon, where friendly bacteria break it down to smaller compounds. Although these compounds are actually vital to good colon health, the process produces some gas.

Gas in the colon is easy to see with an X-ray. Doctors have known for years that there is little relationship between the amount of gas seen in the colon and the sensation of gassiness. Your system absorbs most of the gas your colon produces without your sensing it. What causes feelings of flatulence is not gas per se—the presence of gas in the colon is normal—but rather heightened sensitivity of the colon to gas. In other words, your colon is *irritable* to begin with.

If you already eat lots of fresh fruits and vegetables, gassiness is unlikely to be a problem. You can usually avoid it simply by gradually increasing your fiber intake. If gassiness continues to bother you, your colon is probably hypersensitive. Indeed, irritable colon syndrome, otherwise known as irritable bowel syndrome, or IBS, is the most common intestinal complaint of modern humans. It causes abdominal cramps, gassiness, and alternating constipation and diarrhea. Irritable bowel syndrome is purely the result of our dietary lack of *insoluble* fiber. You can usually relieve it by increasing the amount of insoluble fiber in your diet.

Although soluble fiber works best for lowering blood sugar, insoluble fiber has uniquely beneficial effects on intestinal function. It restores coordination of intestinal muscular contractions, reduces pressure buildup in the intestine, promotes regular bowel movements, disperses gas bubbles, and relieves uncomfortable gassiness. As discussed earlier, the best source of insoluble fiber in the American diet is wheat bran—the husks of wheat kernels—and the best way to get it is to eat bran cereal. A daily bowl of all-bran cereal for a couple of weeks will usually eliminate symptoms of IBS.

Because bran is made from the husks of wheat kernels, there's enough starch in it to push the limits of glycemic load. The glycemic load of a ¹/₂ cup is about the same as that of a slice of white bread. Nevertheless, its beneficial effects on bowel function are probably worth the mild blood sugar surge it might cause.

Whole grain bread is not a particularly good source of insoluble fiber. One slice provides approximately 2 grams of fiber, while ¹/₂ cup of bran cereal delivers 12 grams.

Because bran actually activates and energizes your colon, if your colon is irritable to begin with, you might experience increased cramps and bloating for a few days after you start eating it. These symptoms usually disappear in 2 to 3 days. You can avoid them if you start slowly—perhaps with ¹/₄ cup a day and working your way up to ¹/₂ cup over a week.

Raisin bran and 40 percent bran cereal don't relieve IBS symptoms as well as all-bran cereal does; that's because they contain enough refined flour to negate the benefits of the bran, and their glycemic loads are much too high.

Age: 63

Height: 5' 4"

Pounds lost: 12

Inches lost: 7

Major accomplishment: Brought down her cholesterol by more than 60 points!

Favorite sugar blockers: Peanuts and American cheese

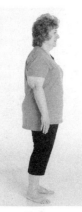

before

JOAN GIANDOMENICO

A Mother's Lesson from Mother Nature

JOAN GIANDOMENICO WAS GROWING FRUS-TRATED with weight loss programs—she was putting in the time and not seeing the desired results. "I exercised 20 minutes, three or four times a week. I tried Weight Watchers and Jenny Craig," she said. But the weight wouldn't budge.

Already struggling with high blood pressure and weight problems—not to mention a family history of type 2 diabetes—Joan knew she had to find a program to help her discover her healthy place. And this time, one that would work.

She heard about the Sugar Blockers Diet through her son Jeremy, who was also participating. Joan had spent many years worrying that Jeremy was following in the footsteps of his father, who suffered from diabetes and had had a heart attack—issues that Joan did not want her son to have to deal with, too. By joining with him, Joan was serving as a companion in the program to help Jeremy stay focused and reach his goals. She was also getting herself on track toward a healthier lifestyle and looking to drop some weight. "I had broken 200 [pounds], and I don't ever want to see it again," she said. As it turns out, she probably won't. While Jeremy's health measures significantly improved, Joan soared in her own success on this program.

Throughout the program, Joan said she kept asking Jeremy about his sugar count. And before they knew it, it became a family affair! "My husband kept telling me '. . . but you're not diabetic,'" Joan said. She knew better, and told him that if she had kept up the lifestyle she had been leading, she very well could have been. Pretty soon, even her husband started to lose weight and notice his pants getting loose around the waist, because Joan was cooking sugar-blocking meals that the whole family enjoyed.

As the weeks passed, Joan's postmeal blood sugar levels went down, and she also found herself feeling more satisfied after meals—and less hungry in between. "I wasn't hungry with this [program]," she said, adding, "I really don't care for sweets too much anymore. If you put a piece of cake in front of me now, I think I would shy away from it."

Joan also finds herself looking forward to exercise. If a brisk walk is all she has time for, a brisk walk is what she takes, and the results still show. After a short stint of treadmill use, Joan was seeing results far bigger than breaking weight loss goals—her overall health was improving. "I had had a problem with a torn meniscus in my knee and couldn't even use the incline on the treadmill," she said. "Now I'm up to 5," she added with a smile. And that's not the only benefit that dropping pounds has had on Joan's life: "I'm getting compliments at work, wearing clothes that I haven't worn for quite a while."

Joan plans to continue the Sugar Blockers Diet and looks forward to reaching new heights in health improvement and weight loss success.

after

7

ACTIVATING YOUR BODY'S **SUGAR-BLOCKING SYSTEMS**

YOUR BODY is a food-processing factory. It converts raw material to energy and structures and stores what's left over. Like any factory, it is capable of handling only a given amount of raw material at a time. Think of your digestive tract as a conveyer belt. The speed that nutrients travel through it must be regulated; otherwise, you overwhelm your system's ability to handle the load.

As you learned in Chapter 4, your body has several ways of regulating how fast nutrients enter your bloodstream. Your pyloric valve, a muscular ring between your stomach and small intestine, is supposed to control how quickly food passes through your digestive tract. However, starch and sugar get absorbed so fast that they never get far enough down your digestive tract to reach the parts of your intestine that send feedback messages to your pyloric valve. Consequently, it doesn't get the message to close off. To make matters worse, the stomachs of overweight people and patients with type 2 diabetes empty faster than normal. Using radioactively labeled food to measure the speed of stomach emptying, University of Texas researchers reported in the *Journal of Nuclear Medicine* that subjects with diabetes emptied their stomachs twice as fast after eating as nondiabetic subjects.

Another line of defense against overly rapid absorption of nutrients is the amount of enzymes your intestinal tract produces. The more amylase you produce, the faster carbohydrates are broken down and absorbed into your bloodstream. Starch is so easy to digest that your digestive tract produces more enzymes than you need, which causes refined carbs to be broken down and absorbed more quickly than other foods.

Your liver is an important sugar blocker. It filters all the blood coming from your intestine. One of the liver's jobs is to remove glucose from your blood after you eat and put it back into your blood between meals. This serves as a sugar "shock absorber," reducing fluctuations of blood sugar, and this dampening function is one of the first things that go awry as you start down the road to diabetes. Instead of taking up glucose after you eat, the liver keeps releasing it, which raises after-meal blood sugar levels.

When you eat, the sooner your beta cells secrete insulin, the less of it you need to keep your blood sugar down. Thus, your beta cells have a special stash of insulin ready to be released as soon as they detect glucose in your system—even before it hits your bloodstream. This early burst of insulin is called the first-phase response. It acts as a sugar blocker of sorts because it decreases the amount of insulin you need to keep your blood sugar down after eating.

As you will see, you can use different foods and eating strategies to take advantage of and bolster all of these natural sugar-blocking mechanisms. There are ways to activate your pyloric valve and slow stomach emptying. You can take measures to reduce the speed with which enzymes break down starch to sugar. In addition, there are things you can do to help your liver take up glucose after you eat, and you can heighten your first-phase insulin response to carbohydrates that you eat. This chapter will show you how you can harness your body's own sugar-blocking systems to soften after-meal blood sugar spikes and reduce its demands for insulin.

If your diet is already low in refined carbohydrates—if you manage to keep your daily glycemic load less than 500—you can use these strategies to make a good diet even better. On those occasions when you splurge a little on starches, the strategies will help lower the glycemic load to an acceptable level.

If you have diabetes that is reasonably well controlled, most of your abnormal blood sugar levels occur after meals. Sugar blockers will help normalize them. Keep in mind, however, that sugar blockers only reduce after-meal blood sugar surges; they don't eliminate them completely. If you pig out on refined carbs, your levels can still shoot up too high.

● ACTIVATING YOUR PYLORIC VALVE: FAT BEFORE YOUR MEAL

As I discussed in Chapter 5, fat is not the culprit it was once made out to be. It's nutritious and satisfying, and it does not raise blood sugar or insulin levels. It's also a natural sugar blocker. Consuming even a small amount of fat 10 to 30 minutes before a meal can lower after-meal blood sugar levels by as much as 38 percent. It does this by slowing stomach emptying.

Your small intestine is highly sensitive to the presence of fat. As soon as a small amount reaches your intestine, it triggers a reflex that shuts off the pyloric valve and slows digestion. It also stimulates a nerve pathway that helps your liver perform its shock-absorber function. It takes remarkably little fat to have this effect. While you need a full serving or more of fruit or vegetables to inhibit starch absorption, just a teaspoon of fat—easily provided by a handful of nuts, a piece of cheese, a slice of bacon, or some oil in a salad dressing—will slow stomach emptying.

Although any kind of fat will blunt sugar spikes, some types of fat have been shown to have other health benefits as well. Food scientists divide fats into two categories: saturated and unsaturated. You can tell them apart by looking at them. Saturated fats are solid at room temperature; unsaturated fats are liquids. Like cholesterol, saturated fats were once thought to contribute to obesity and heart disease, but that theory has been disproven. An analysis of 21 studies, recently published in the *American Journal of Clinical Nutrition,* indicated that there is no significant evidence that saturated fat increases the risk of heart disease.

Among unsaturated fats, there are two kinds that have particularly beneficial effects on the heart and blood vessels: monounsaturated fatty acids, or MUFAs, and omega-3 fatty acids.

Monounsaturated Fatty Acids

As with any fat, if you consume a small amount of olive oil before a meal, it will slow stomach emptying. However, olive oil has other healthful qualities. Of the foods we commonly eat, olive oil is the richest in MUFAs. Besides their sugar-blocking effects, these good fats improve the balance between good and bad cholesterol. In one Pennsylvania State University study, high-MUFA diets lowered LDL cholesterol by 14 percent, triglyceride levels by 13 percent, and total cholesterol by 10 percent. These fatty acids also lower blood pressure. Several research studies have linked olive oil consumption to reduced risk of heart disease.

Nuts and avocados also contain generous amounts of MUFAs, as do olives themselves, of course. Nut oils, canola oil, safflower oil, and, best of all, dark chocolate are also good sources of MUFAs.

Omega-3 Fatty Acids

Your body needs many different types of fats to make membranes, hormones, and other important structures. It can convert whatever fat is available to most of the kinds of fats you need. However, there are a few fats your system cannot produce. Because it is *essential* that you get them from your diet, these fats are called "essential" fatty acids.

One essential fatty acid that is particularly hard to come by is a type called omega-3. The main sources of omega-3s in nature are grasses and leaves, which we generally don't eat. Humans have historically gotten their omega-3s by eating animals that do eat grasses and leaves, including cattle, sheep, and poultry. The problem is that in recent years, less of the meat we eat comes from grazing animals and more from livestock kept in feedlots and fed grain, which is largely devoid of omega-3s. Although meat and eggs still provide some omega-3s, our diet contains significantly less than that of our ancestors.

Free-range beef and chicken products contain more omega-3s because they come from animals that graze on grass and leaves. The flesh of certain coldwater fish—including salmon, anchovies, mackerel, herring, and sardines—contains high concentrations of omega-3 fatty acids, which fish get from feeding on algae.

Omega-3s reduce blood triglyceride levels, stabilize the electrical activity of the heart, and counteract inflammation. They also improve your body's sensitivity to insulin, which reduces insulin demands.

Besides eating more omega-3–rich foods, a good way to increase the omega-3 content of your diet is to take a fish oil supplement. You can buy capsules of fish oil at most pharmacies. As a source of fat, fish oil taken before a meal can also serve as a sugar blocker. The usual daily dose is two or three capsules, each of which contains about 1 gram of oil. That isn't quite enough for effective sugar blocking—research has shown that it takes about 5 grams of fat to reduce after-meal blood sugar levels. However, you don't need to take the same amount every day. If the meal you're about to eat contains starch, you can take five capsules beforehand and then skip the next day's dose if you want.

Nuts: How Natural Can You Get?

If your definition of a "natural" food is one that humans have been eating for a long time, then nuts are as natural as you can get. They're the oldest-known plant part that humans eat. Nuts have been a significant part of the human diet since prehistoric times.

In the past, when fat had a bad name, nuts puzzled researchers because, despite their high fat content, studies showed that people who ate a lot of them ended up with less heart disease than people who didn't. Actually, this is not surprising, considering that nuts are full of healthy stuff, including protein, MUFAs, omega-3 fatty acids, and fiber, and they contain little starch or sugar. They are the perfect snack for someone trying to cut carbs: They'll satisfy your hunger and provide vital nutrients, and they won't raise your blood sugar or insulin levels even a bit.

Nuts also have sugar-blocking powers. A few handfuls as an appetizer before a starch-containing meal will reduce your after-meal blood sugar and insulin levels. Researchers at the Clinical Nutrition and Risk Factor Modification Centre at St. Michael's Hospital in Toronto reported in the journal *Metabolism* that eating 60 grams of nuts (about two handfuls) with 50 grams of white bread (2 slices) will result in a blood sugar surge that is 37 percent lower than the surge produced by eating the bread alone. If you have three handfuls, it will reduce the blood sugar rise by 55 percent. Peanuts and walnuts have the same effect on blood sugar; it's probably true of all nuts. As test panelist Tammy Hobar noted, "Eating almonds while I cook dinner is twofold: It's a sugar blocker, but it also helps me eat less at dinner."

In addition to acting as a sugar blocker, nuts lower blood levels of bad cholesterol and raise good cholesterol levels. Numerous research studies have linked nut consumption to reduced risk of heart and blood vessel disease.

Sugar-Blocking Flours

If you like baked goods—breads, muffins, cookies, etc.—but are trying to cut out starch, you might think you're out of luck, but that's not necessarily so. A good cook can make delicious low-starch baked items using non-starch flours, usually made of nuts or seeds, such as almond, walnut, or pumpkin-seed flour.

As tasty as nonstarch flours can be in their own right, their flavor and texture are different from their regular wheat-flour counterparts—not necessarily worse or better, just different. However, you don't need to eliminate wheat flour altogether to keep the glycemic load of baked goods in an acceptable range. Adding nuts and nut flour to regular flour will reduce the glycemic load of whatever regular flour you include in a recipe. For example, if you combine wheat flour with an equal portion of nuts or nut flour, not only do you cut in half the wheat flour content of the baked good, but the starch-blocking effect of the nuts will also reduce the glycemic load of the remaining wheat flour by an additional third. That means you reduce the glycemic load by 66 percent. In Chapter 9 you'll find more information on baking with nut flours, along with more than 50 delicious recipes, including Green Banana–Nut Bread and Nutty Brownies.

Cinnamon

Two teaspoons of cinnamon will lower your blood sugar response to a serving of carbohydrate by 13 percent. That's not much, but the effect lasts for at least 12 hours. Several studies have shown that regular consumption of cinnamon improves long-term diabetes control.

Cinnamon reduces blood sugar by triggering intestinal hormones that delay stomach emptying and improve insulin efficiency. The trouble is, the foods that most folks add cinnamon to—oatmeal, cookies, pie—are starches. However, if you absolutely must have some toast or rice, and you like it with cinnamon, it might help a little.

● RESTORING ENZYME BALANCE: VINEGAR

In the past, adherents of folk medicine thought that vinegar could cure an assortment of ills—stomachaches, croup, heart disease, and even poison ivy. Physicians also used it for years to treat diabetes before insulin became available. Although most claims of vinegar's healing powers are baseless, it turns out that it is actually an effective starch blocker. Taking a couple of tablespoons before you eat starch reduces after-meal blood sugar levels by as much as 64 percent—comparable to the effects of prescription starch blockers.

And you don't have to have diabetes to benefit. Vinegar works well for reducing blood sugar surges and taming insulin demands for people without diabetes who are insulin resistant, which includes most overweight individuals and prediabetics.

Scientists attribute vinegar's starch-blocking powers to its high acetic acid content. It's not just the acidity that blocks starch—other acids don't have the same effect. Acetic acid deactivates amylase, the enzyme that breaks down starch to sugar. This explains why vinegar has no effect on the absorption of sugar, only starch. In other words, vinegar won't help your blood sugar if you eat candy, but it can help if you eat bread.

In addition to inhibiting starch absorption, vinegar increases the body's sensitivity to insulin, which further reduces insulin demands and promotes weight loss. Studies have shown that vinegar taken with a meal lessens hunger for hours afterward.

You should consume vinegar immediately upon starting your meal. You can take advantage of its starch-blocking powers by drinking an ounce (2 tablespoons) in a glass of water before a meal. A bigger dose, up to 5 tablespoons, is more effective at inhibiting starch absorption but could give you acid indigestion. A tastier way, though, is to put it in a salad dressing or sprinkle it on food. Vinegar makes a good condiment, bringing out the flavor of food as salt does. You can sprinkle it on a salad, meat, or vegetables, or you can add it to an olive oil bread dip. But remember, for it to work as a starch blocker, you need to take it before eating starch, not afterward.

Pickles

Research has shown that consuming a full-size cucumber pickle before eating starch significantly reduces the after-meal blood sugar level. That's not surprising, considering that pickles are full of vinegar and soluble fiber. If you're not in the mood for a pickle, you can create the same effect by slicing up cucumbers and pouring vinegar on them—an old favorite. You've heard that pickles contain a lot of salt? Don't worry. Recent studies

---

WHITE Beans Revisited

A S MENTIONED in Chapter 4, food scientists have known for years that a substance in white beans called phaseolamin is a potent inhibitor of the digestive enzyme amylase—at least in the test tube. You won't get enough of it to block the digestion of starch from eating white beans, though; there just isn't enough of it in a serving of beans to do the job. And even when white bean powder was sold as an aid to weight loss, it didn't work. The problem is that stomach acid deactivates most of the phaseolamin before it gets to the intestine. (It's possible that antacid medication would make phaseolamin work better, though researchers haven't tested that theory.)

Manufacturers have recently developed a more concentrated form of white bean extract called Phase 2, which works better than the old preparations did. One study showed that subjects who consumed a dose of Phase 2 with bread had a subsequent glucose spike that was 34 percent lower than if they'd eaten bread alone. Phase 2 works best in powder form—sprinkled directly on starch—rather than swallowed in capsules beforehand.

indicate that, contrary to previous beliefs, dietary salt is not what causes high blood pressure. (See Chapter 9 for a simple Cucumber and Vinegar Salad—plus some easy vinaigrettes that you can use on salads or over vegetables.)

● SYNCHRONIZING YOUR LIVER AND YOUR GUT: ALCOHOL

Alcohol contains calories, but it won't raise your blood sugar. Wine and hard liquor have negligible glycemic loads because most of the sugar in them has been fermented away. Beer contains some sugar, so its glycemic load is higher—the glycemic load of a 12-ounce glass is approximately 60 percent of that of a slice of white bread.

It turns out that alcohol has unique sugar-blocking properties. Here's how it works: Your liver normally converts some of the fat and protein in your blood to glucose, and that's added to the glucose you eat. Alcohol consumed with a meal temporarily halts your liver's glucose production and reduces its contribution to after-meal blood sugar elevations. Thus, a glass of beer or wine or a shot of hard liquor consumed before a meal will reduce the glycemic load of a typical serving of starch by approximately 25 percent.

Of course, that doesn't mean you should consume several drinks. Remember that calories consumed in liquids tend to add to, rather than take the place of, the calories in solid foods. Drinking an alcoholic beverage before a meal will not reduce the amount you eat. In fact, alcohol delays the sensation of fullness from eating. Too much alcohol piles on calories and makes you tend to overeat. Also, cocktails made with sugar-sweetened mixers such as ginger ale and tonic have high glycemic loads and will raise your blood sugar. Nevertheless, if you're accustomed to having a glass of wine or beer with your meals and it doesn't cause you to overeat, it can actually help keep your blood sugar and insulin levels down. Research suggests that drinking an ounce or two of alcohol daily reduces the risk of diabetes and heart disease. "I love that I could still have wine," said test panelist Jane Wilchak. "That was nice."

● MAKING INSULIN MORE EFFICIENT: PROTEIN WITH CARBS

Most of the protein in our diets comes from animal products—eggs, meat, and dairy products—although we get some from legumes such as beans and peas. Protein is the main component of most of the tissues of your body—muscles, blood, internal organs, and enzymes. You can't live without it.

Just as the building block of carbohydrates is glucose, the building block of protein is a type of molecule called amino acid. There are 20 different amino acids, 10 of which are "essential"—you need to get them from your diet because your body doesn't make them.

Researchers have found that a serving of protein consumed with starch can reduce the subsequent blood sugar surge by as much as 44 percent. It does this by causing your beta cells to secrete insulin.

You probably like the idea that protein can lower your blood sugar, but you probably wish it wouldn't do it by causing your beta cells to secrete more insulin. After all, you're trying to reduce the amount of insulin that your body has to make. However, protein makes your beta cells secrete insulin *sooner* after you eat than if you'd consumed carbohydrates alone— the first-phase insulin response. As you'll recall, the sooner your beta cells secrete insulin after you eat carbohydrates, the less of it you need to keep your blood sugar down. In other words, protein consumed with carbohydrates causes insulin to act more efficiently, which ultimately reduces the amount of insulin needed.

AN AFTER-MEAL Stroll

QUESTION: How can you stop a glucose spike after it starts?

Answer: Go for a 20-minute walk.

As mentioned in Chapter 4, the main reason exercise is so important for losing weight and preventing or treating diabetes is that it sensitizes muscles to insulin. This effect lasts for 24 to 48 hours. However, there's another way that exercise can lower your blood sugar. The contraction of muscles instantly opens up channels in your muscle cells, which allows them to take up glucose *independent of insulin.* These channels open when your muscles start contracting and close when they stop. University of Wisconsin researchers have found that a 20-minute walk immediately following a carbohydrate-containing meal cuts the after-meal blood sugar surge *in half.*

So if you slip up and eat something you shouldn't, get up and go for a walk. Better yet, make it a habit.

● A ROUGH SCIENCE

As you can see, the effects of carbohydrates on blood sugar levels are not as straightforward as once believed. It's not as simple as "a carb is a carb." Different carbohydrates can have different effects on your blood sugar levels even if they deliver the same amounts of glucose into your bloodstream. That's why the glycemic loads of carbohydrates vary so much.

As useful as the glycemic load tables are, you should realize that these measurements are frustratingly imprecise. They drive scientists crazy because they vary so much among research studies and among individuals. How high your blood sugar and insulin levels rise after you eat a carbohydrate is influenced by the foods you consume with it, the order in which you eat them, and your activities before and after meals, all of which need to be taken into account when you're measuring glycemic load. The only way to tell for sure how much a particular food or combination of

THE IDEAL Eating Style

SCIENTISTS HAVE STUDIED dozens of different diets, and while much controversy remains as to what constitutes an ideal eating style, some themes have emerged. As it turns out, the diets that have been most consistently associated with reduced risk of diabetes and heart disease are ones that contain plenty of natural sugar blockers.

An example is what's known as the Mediterranean diet, which the American Heart Association now recommends as a healthy eating style. This way of eating resembles the customary diets of Italy and Greece, including Crete. Traditionally, the inhabitants of those countries ate plenty of fat and cholesterol, but they also consumed more fruit, vegetables, nuts, olive oil, vinegar, salads, and wine than Americans do—all foods that inhibit the absorption of starch. In one large European study, adherence to this eating pattern reduced diabetes and heart disease rates by more than half.

Actually, Americans eat those foods, too, just not as much or as consistently as the Greeks and Italians do. By cutting out as much starch as you can and consuming lots of natural starch blockers, chances are you will enjoy the same benefits.

---

food and sugar blockers will raise your blood sugar is to measure it before and after you eat.

If the glycemic load is a rough science, you might call sugar blocking a black art. It's hard to predict how much any sugar blocker or combination of sugar blockers will lower your blood sugar. However, scientists have found that the effects of a certain food on blood sugar are more predictable when measured in the same individual in the same setting. If you measure your after-meal blood sugar and find that a particular combination of sugar blockers and food works for you a couple of times, it will probably work for you again.

One way of dealing with the unpredictability of sugar blockers is to combine them. If one sugar blocker has less of a blood sugar–lowering effect for you than predicted, another might have more of an effect. Also, as I mentioned in Chapter 4, their sugar-blocking effects add up—especially if they act on different parts of the digestive process at once. For example, researchers have found that combining soluble fiber, a "sponge"-type sugar blocker, with vinegar, an enzyme inhibitor, reduces after-meal blood sugar more than doubling the amount of either sugar blocker alone. In Part III you'll learn several ways to combine sugar blockers.

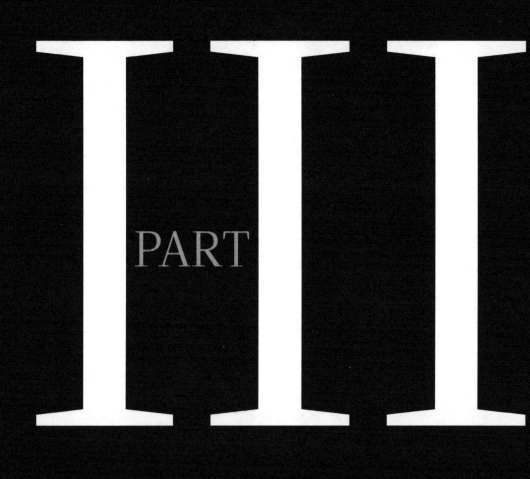

PART III

THE SUGAR
BLOCKERS DIET

O N THE FIRST PAGE of Chapter 1, I said that it doesn't matter if you're a strict vegetarian, a voracious carnivore, or an incurable chocoholic. The important thing is that you block sugar. Now you understand why: Eating fat is not what makes you fat. Eating cholesterol does not cause high blood cholesterol. Carbohydrates per se are not the problem. The problem is carbs that are absorbed into your bloodstream too quickly. If your diet is typical, you squander most of the insulin that your beta cells make on after-meal blood sugar spikes. Excessive insulin production makes you fat and wears out your insulin-making cells.

If your goal is to lose weight and prevent diabetes and heart disease, the evidence is in: It does no good to avoid eggs, meat, dairy products, or fatty plant products such as nuts, olives, and avocados. Nor should you avoid "good carbs" like fresh fruits and vegetables. In fact, you can even have a few "bad carbs." *You just need to make sure the carbohydrates you eat trickle into your bloodstream slowly and don't rush in all at once.*

The next chapter will show you how to fit sugar blockers into your regular eating patterns. Chapter 9 puts sugar blockers to work in the kitchen and includes more than 50 delicious recipes. And in Chapter 10, you'll learn how to use sugar-blocking techniques in real-life situations.

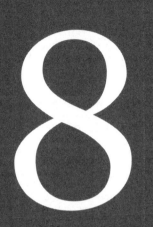

8

PUTTING
THE PLAN
INTO **ACTION**

NOW THAT YOU HAVE LEARNED about the effects of different foods on your blood sugar, it's time to put the information to work. The plan is simple: Identify the foods that cause sugar shocks, avoid them when you can, and block them when you can't. Our testers loved how easy it was to follow this plan: Cindy Swan, who lost 10 pounds in 6 weeks on the plan, remarked, "I felt like I wasn't doing it right because it was so easy. You can eat anything!" Valerie Hayes, who lost 18½ pounds, agreed: "I found it really easy to do and I liked that. I didn't really feel like I was trying that much."

Here's how you do it.

● STEP 1: IDENTIFY THE CULPRITS

There are only two kinds of foods you need to worry about: starch and sugar-containing beverages.

Starches are easy to identify. Because of starch's physical properties and the way we customarily prepare it, it is never blended into other foods. It stands right out in the open. You can spot the culprits from across the room. The main offenders are bread and other baked goods, potatoes, rice, pasta, and breakfast cereals.

If you're at all concerned about your weight or your blood sugar, you know you shouldn't drink nondiet sodas. However, keep in mind that fruit juices—orange, apple, grapefruit, and cranberry juice—are also sugar-containing beverages, even without added sugar.

That's it. You don't need to try to avoid fat, cholesterol, salt, or trans fats. You don't even need to try to reduce calories. Just focus on eliminating refined carbohydrates.

In case you're unsure of who the culprits are, here's a complete list.

Any kind of grain, including:

- Barley
- Buckwheat
- Millet
- Oats
- Quinoa
- Rice (white, brown, and wild)
- Rye
- Wheat

Foods that are made of grain:

- Bagels
- Bread (white, brown, and whole grain)
- Cakes, cookies, brownies, cupcakes
- Cereal, granola
- Chips, crackers, pretzels
- Doughnuts, muffins, croissants, pastries
- Oatmeal
- Pancakes, crepes, waffles

- Pasta, couscous
- Piecrust
- Pitas, tortillas, wraps
- Pizza crust

Potatoes and potato products:

- Potato chips
- Potato pancakes
- Red potatoes
- Sweet potatoes
- White potatoes

Corn and corn products:

- Cornbread, corn tortillas
- Corn chips
- Corn on the cob
- Grits

Sugar-sweetened beverages:

- Energy drinks
- Fruit juice
- Regular soda
- Slushies and smoothies

● STEP 2: AVOID THE CULPRITS WHEN YOU CAN

As discussed in Chapter 5, your risk of obesity and diabetes begins to increase when your daily glycemic load exceeds approximately 500. Here's a simple way to ensure that your starch intake stays in the safe zone: Figure that the glycemic loads of the *nonstarchy* carbohydrates—the fresh fruits and vegetables—in a typical day add up to about 250. You've seen that the glycemic load of a typical serving of starch ranges around 250. That means if you don't eat more than *one typical serving of starch a day*, your daily glycemic load shouldn't exceed 500. You can eat a full serving once a day, a half serving twice a day, or a third of a serving three times a day.

How large is a typical serving? An amount that would fill about a quarter of a normal-size dinner plate. Here are some examples.

- 2 slices of bread
- 1 medium potato
- 1 ear of corn
- 1 cup of pasta or rice
- 1 cup of cereal
- 1 medium bagel or roll

● STEP 3: USE SUGAR BLOCKERS WHEN YOU CAN'T AVOID STARCHES

Starch is cheap filler food. It's foisted upon us at every turn. You can't always avoid it (and sometimes you don't want to!). However, as you've seen, there are many foods that blunt its effects on your blood sugar. How do you fit them into your everyday eating patterns?

As it turns out, the way we Americans customarily structure our meals—when we take the time to relax and enjoy them—actually provides an excellent framework for putting sugar-blocking techniques into action. Consider the following opportunities to slow the breakdown of starch and its absorption into your bloodstream.

▶ We frequently have an appetizer before our meal, which provides an occasion for eating a fatty snack. As discussed in Chapter 7, a small amount of fat consumed before a meal activates your pyloric valve and slows stomach emptying.

▶ We often eat a salad and a serving of vegetables with our meals, both of which provide soluble fiber. In Chapter 6 you learned that soluble fiber slows stomach emptying, soaks up glucose, and delays the absorption of glucose into your bloodstream.

▶ We often use vinegar-based salad dressings. As discussed in Chapter 7, vinegar partially deactivates amylase, the enzyme responsible for breaking down starch into sugar.

▶ We usually include a source of protein—meat, fish, or poultry—with our meals. In Chapters 4 and 7 you learned that protein consumed with starch triggers a first-phase insulin response, which improves insulin's efficiency so that you need less of it to keep your blood sugar down.

▶ Some of us have a glass of wine with meals, which helps the liver remove sugar from the bloodstream after eating.

▶ We save our dessert for last. If we slip up and have a little too much sugar for dessert, the sugar blockers we had with our meal help keep it from raising our blood sugar.

▶ Some of us even go for an after-meal stroll, which, as discussed in Chapter 7, allows our muscles to remove sugar from the bloodstream without the need for insulin.

There you are—an eating pattern that lets you combine several sugar blockers while conforming to the way we customarily eat. When you eat starch with a meal, try to do the following:

1. Have a fatty snack 10 to 30 minutes before your meal.
2. Start your meal with a salad.

3. Use a vinegar-based dressing.

4. Include a serving of vegetables with your meal.

5. Include protein with your meal.

6. Consider having a glass of wine or a shot of alcohol with your meal.

7. Eat sweets for dessert only.

8. Go for a walk afterward.

And most important of all, never eat refined carbohydrates on an empty stomach. Of course, it may not be realistic for you to incorporate all of those sugar blockers with every meal. But remember that combining sugar blockers works better than relying on just one kind. As a rule of thumb, use three types of sugar blockers for each serving of starch.

How Much Does It Take?

You need only a little fat to slow stomach emptying. Five grams—about a teaspoon—will do. A handful of nuts or cheese easily provides that. It takes 2 to 4 tablespoons of vinegar to slow starch absorption—about as much as you would normally put on a typical serving of salad. A modest serving of protein—say, 4 ounces—will boost the first-phase insulin response to starch. It takes about 1½ ounces of alcohol, approximately the amount in a typical-size glass of wine or cocktail, to reduce your after-meal blood sugar.

Fiber is another matter. You need a lot of it to do the job. It takes 10 grams—about two large servings of high-fiber fruits or vegetables—to reduce your after-meal blood sugar surge by 25 percent. Most fruits, vegetables, nuts, and seeds contain soluble fiber. However, keep in mind that the balance of fiber to sugar content is also important. The best foods to use for sugar blocking are those that are not only high in fiber but that have glycemic loads of less than 50. Here's a handy list of low-glycemic load fiber sources, in order of fiber content.

FOOD	SERVING SIZE	FIBER (GRAMS)	ESTIMATED GLYCEMIC LOAD
FRUITS			
Raspberries	1 cup	8.4	30
Blackberries (raw)	1 cup	7.6	Less than 15
Strawberries	1 cup	3.8	30
Avocado	½ avocado	3.5	20
Papaya, cubed	1 cup	2.5	30
Apricots	3 apricots	2.4	24
Grapefruit	½ grapefruit	1.4	32
VEGETABLES			
Artichoke (cooked)	1 cup	9.1	Less than 15
Sauerkraut	1 cup	5.9	Less than 15
Collard greens	1 cup	5.3	Less than 15
Carrot (cooked)	1 cup	5.1	Less than 15
Turnip greens (cooked)	1 cup	5	Less than 15
Broccoli	1 cup	4.5	Less than 15
Spinach (cooked)	1 cup	4.3	Less than 15
Brussels sprouts	1 cup	4.1	40
Okra (cooked)	1 cup	4	Less than 15
String beans	1 cup	4	Less than 15
Cabbage (cooked)	1 cup	3.5	Less than 15
Mushrooms (cooked)	1 cup	3.4	Less than 15
Cauliflower	1 cup	3.3	Less than 15
Turnips	1 cup	3.1	20
Dandelion greens	1 cup	3	Less than 15
Peppers (red)	1 cup	3	Less than 15
Asparagus	1 cup	2.9	Less than 15
Onions (cooked)	1 cup	2.9	Less than 15
Mustard greens (cooked)	1 cup	2.8	Less than 15

(continued)

FOOD	SERVING SIZE	FIBER (GRAMS)	ESTIMATED GLYCEMIC LOAD
VEGETABLES *(continued)*			
Peppers (green)	1 cup	2.7	Less than 15
Scallions	1 cup	2.6	Less than 15
Eggplant	1 cup	2.5	Less than 15
Carrot (raw)	7½" carrot	2.2	Less than 15
Lettuce, looseleaf	2 cups	2.2	Less than 15
Celery (diced)	1 cup	2	Less than 15
Lettuce, romaine	2 cups	2	Less than 15
Tomatoes (chopped)	1 cup	2	Less than 15
Bean sprouts	1 cup	1.9	Less than 15
Water chestnuts	½ cup	1.8	Less than 15
Cucumber pickle	1 large	1.6	Less than 15
Lettuce, iceberg	2 cups	1.6	Less than 15
Spinach (raw)	2 cups	1.6	Less than 15
Onions (raw)	½ cup	1.5	Less than 15
Lettuce, butterhead	2 cups	1.1	Less than 15
Alfalfa sprouts	1 cup	0.8	Less than 15
Cucumber (peeled)	1 cup	0.8	Less than 15
Mushrooms (raw)	1 cup	0.8	Less than 15
BEANS AND LEGUMES			
Lentils	½ cup	7.8	30
Soybeans	1 cup	7.6	Less than 15
Beans, pinto	½ cup	7.4	45
Beans, lima	½ cup	6.6	34
Beans, kidney	½ cup	6.5	30
Chickpeas	½ cup	6.2	45

FOOD	SERVING SIZE	FIBER (GRAMS)	ESTIMATED GLYCEMIC LOAD
BEANS AND LEGUMES (continued)			
Beans, navy	½ cup	5.8	45
Peas	½ cup	2.3	32
NUTS AND SEEDS			
Chia seeds	1 Tbsp	5.5	Less than 15
Almonds	24 nuts	3.2	Less than 15
Sunflower seeds	¼ cup	2.9	Less than 15
Hazelnuts	20 nuts	2.7	Less than 15
Peanuts	28 nuts	2.3	Less than 15
Walnuts	14 halves	1.9	Less than 15
Cashews	18 nuts	0.6	28
FIBER SUPPLEMENTS			
Psyllium husks	1 Tbsp	4.5	Less than 15
Oat bran (raw)	¼ cup	3.7	Less than 15
Guar gum	1 tsp	3	Less than 15
Metamucil	1 tsp	3	Less than 15

On page 136 is a list of assorted sugar blockers. The amounts listed are the minimum amounts you need for effective sugar blocking.

● HOW TO TELL IF THE PLAN IS WORKING FOR YOU

How high your blood sugar goes after you eat a meal depends on a host of factors: how much you chew your food, particle size, fiber content, protein and fat content, natural enzyme inhibitors, thickness, acidity, physical activities before and after, and even sleep quality and stress. Because so many things can influence after-meal blood sugar levels, it's hard to predict what effect a combination of food and sugar blockers will have on your blood sugar.

SUGAR BLOCKER	AMOUNT	WHEN TO EAT
Cheese	½ oz or 1 Tbsp	10 to 30 minutes before starch
Fish oil capsules	Four 1,200 mg capsules	10 to 30 minutes before starch
Nuts	1 oz or 2 Tbsp	10 to 30 minutes before starch
Oil	1 oz or 2 Tbsp	10 to 30 minutes before starch
Vinegar	2 Tbsp	Before starch
Pickle	1 medium	Before starch
Soluble fiber	10 g (see table on pages 133–135 for specific foods)	Before or with starch
Meat, fish, or poultry	4 oz raw (3 oz cooked)	Before or with starch
Eggs	2 whole	Before or with starch
Milk or yogurt (full-fat)	1 cup	Before or with starch
Chia seeds	2 Tbsp	Before or with starch
Flaxseeds	3 Tbsp	Before or with starch
Wine or beer	5 oz or 1 glass	Before or with starch
Liquor	1½ oz or 1 shot	Before or with starch
Cinnamon	2 tsp	With starch
Phase 2 (white bean extract) powder	2 tsp	Sprinkled on starch

Going to the doctor won't tell you how high your blood sugar rises after you eat a particular kind of food unless you rush in and have your blood sugar checked immediately after eating the food. However, if you have diabetes, you're probably used to measuring your own blood sugar with a glucometer—a portable blood sugar–measuring device. If so, you can see for yourself what various foods and combinations of foods and sugar blockers do to your blood sugar.

You don't have to have diabetes to gain useful information by measuring your blood sugar. Glucometers are helpful if you're just trying to lose weight. You can buy one at any pharmacy and easily teach yourself how to use it.

Some of the test panelists tried this, with eye-opening results. "I never knew what my glucose or anything was, really. [It turned out to be] higher than I thought, but it's come down a lot," said Joan Giandomenico.

You can experiment by checking your blood sugar a few hours after different meals. A reasonable goal is to keep your blood sugar from rising more than 40 points from where it was before you ate. If you have diabetes, you should try to keep your after-meal levels less than 160. Levels of 160 to 200 are okay but not ideal; more than 200 is definitely too high. If you consistently get postmeal blood sugar levels higher than 200, examine your eating and activity patterns to see if you can pinpoint what's causing these highs. (The journal pages in Appendix B can help you do this.)

If you don't have diabetes, a good way to tell how much your blood sugar should rise after meals is to check it a few times after you eat something starchy—say, a few slices of bread or a serving of french fries—and then try to keep your after-meal readings below that level. As with those with diabetes, your blood sugar shouldn't rise more than 40 points 2 to 3 hours after a meal above what it was before.

When you reduce the glycemic load of the carbohydrates you eat and start using sugar blockers, you may notice a paradox: Sometimes your blood sugar level will be lower after you eat than it will be the next morning. The reason is that, instead of rushing into your bloodstream all at once, glucose is still trickling into your bloodstream the following morning. That's a sign that you are, indeed, slowing the absorption of glucose into your bloodstream.

The A1C Test

As discussed in Chapter 3, every time your blood sugar rises, it puts a minuscule coat of sugar on the hemoglobin in your red blood cells, which stays there for up to 3 months. Doctors can measure the amount of sugar on your hemoglobin with a test called hemoglobin A1C, or just A1C. Your A1C level reflects your average blood sugar over the previous 3 months. If your blood sugar is always high, your A1C level will be high. However, if your fasting blood sugar is normal but your A1C level is high, your blood sugar is probably spiking after many of your meals. Indeed, among those with pre-diabetes and diabetes, after-meal blood sugar surges account for as much as 70 percent of abnormal blood sugar levels.

Normally, your A1C level should be less than 6. If it's between 6 and 6.5, your blood sugar is probably okay when you haven't eaten for a while but rising too high after some meals. This is a sign of prediabetes and often progresses to diabetes. An A1C level greater than 6.5 usually means that you have diabetes. Patients with diabetes whose blood sugar levels are poorly controlled often have A1C levels greater than 12.

If you have diabetes, the usual goal is to keep your A1C at less than 7. If your A1C is between 7 and 8, most of the high blood sugar you're having is probably occurring after meals. The way to lower it further—in fact, the only way—is to get rid of after-meal spikes. With an effective sugar-blocking program, you can lower your A1C levels in a month, although it will continue to decline for 3 months.

Mood and Energy

Sometimes you can tell what your blood sugar is doing by how you feel. When you eat something starchy or sugary, your blood sugar shoots up, which causes your beta cells to secrete a large burst of insulin. This some-times causes your blood sugar to fall too fast. Most folks can't feel their blood sugar go up. However, they can often feel it go down. Rapidly falling blood sugar causes weakness, shakiness, poor concentration, and dizzi-ness. Doctors call this reactive hypoglycemia, or low blood sugar.

Blood sugar highs and lows can go on all day, resulting in alternating irritability and fatigue, which can leave you feeling exhausted at the end of the day. You can eliminate these symptoms by avoiding high-glycemic load foods and using sugar blockers to slow the absorption of carbohydrates. "I don't even need to take my blood sugar to know it's going to go up," reported Michelle Newhard. "I tried a piece of cake at breakfast and was grumpy by lunch."

If you use a sugar blocker that slows stomach emptying, you tend to eat less and stay full longer after meals. For example, eating a handful of nuts 10 to 20 minutes before a meal will slow stomach emptying, so you get full faster. Over the course of a few weeks, you may begin to notice that your habits change, you become content with less food at meals, and you lose the urge to snack between meals.

Having a stable blood sugar level reduces your craving for refined carbohydrates. Researchers at the Royal Infirmary of Edinburgh gave subjects insulin shots to produce mild hypoglycemia. The researchers then gave the subjects a choice of several foods and observed which ones they chose to eat. Compared with a group of volunteers that did not get insulin, the hypoglycemic volunteers chose more starchy, sugary foods. In other words, low blood sugar causes a craving for the same kinds of starchy and sugary foods that caused the reaction in the first place. If you get rid of high-glycemic load foods, you'll crave them less.

Women who have irregular periods caused by polycystic ovary syndrome have a built-in mechanism for telling if they're eating right and getting enough exercise. As soon as they reduce their glycemic load and start walking, their periods often become regular again.

One blood test that changes dramatically when you reduce your intake of rapidly absorbed carbohydrates is your blood triglyceride level. Within a few days, it will drop like a rock. As discussed in Chapter 2, high triglyceride levels lead to lower levels of good cholesterol. If you lower your triglyceride level, after a few weeks your good cholesterol levels will rise.

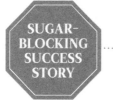
Age: 52

Height: 5' 7"

Pounds lost: 17½

Inches lost: 13¾

**Major
accomplishment:**
Double-digit weight
loss and 2¼" off
her waist!

**Favorite
sugar blockers:**
Pecans, Jarlsberg
cheese, cucumber
salad with vinegar

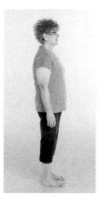

before

LINDA FREY
A Lesson in Smart Snacking

LINDA FREY HAD ALWAYS RESORTED to sugary, carb-laden snacks for comfort and quick hunger fixes, but her extra weight began to pile on when her mom got sick. Suddenly Linda found her schedule somersaulting out of balance. She would leave work to go straight to the hospital to visit her dying mother without taking time to attend to her own needs, dietary or otherwise.

"I would get home around 8:30 and eat carbs—like cereal, mac and cheese, pretzels, macaroni salad, and tortilla chips," she said. Those snack foods were Linda's main source of nutrition before she started the Sugar Blockers Diet, but she knew she'd have to change her eating habits to get her body and her health back on track.

On the plan, Linda traded in chips and pretzels for high-protein snacks like cheeses and nuts—and she couldn't have asked for better results. The first 2 weeks felt like a detox as she learned to quell her hunger with raw veggies and her new favorite food: pecans. "I didn't realize that the protein from nuts was so important," she said. "They're a great filler, they taste good, and they make a portable snack." By the end of 2 weeks, she had shed almost 8 pounds.

"I feel more energetic, and I'm not huffing and puffing anymore," Linda reported. "I feel more relaxed, my blood pressure has decreased, and I never thought my cholesterol would drop, but it did . . . even while eating eggs and bacon 4 days a week. People have commented on my less stressed state and how good I look."

The Sugar Blockers Diet works in part because it's so flexible. Linda has strictures in her throat, scar tissue that narrows the passage of her esophagus and makes swallowing certain foods more dangerous. She has found that making suitable substitutions is a cinch. "The strictures limit my eating of meat, so I eat fish in its place. I don't eat lettuce or endive. Instead, I make a salad with chickpeas, raw cucumbers, sunflower seeds, and other toppings."

Linda is also more conscientious about how much starch she eats. She eats a smaller serving of cereal in the morning and leaves much of her pizza crust. "You're never hungry," she said, explaining that when she eats the Sugar Blockers Diet way, she feels full sooner and her fullness lasts longer.

Her biggest surprise has been how easy it is to stay on the plan while dining out. Once Linda lets the servers know that she's on a low-starch program, they avoid placing bread on the table and are quick to recommend low-carb entrées and side dishes. Eating at parties is also surprisingly easy. "I found that hummus is a great party food to use as a dip with raw vegetables."

One thing is certain: Linda will be sticking to the Sugar Blockers Diet long after she reaches her ideal weight. "After those first 2 weeks, there was no looking back. I knew it worked."

after

9

SUGAR-BLOCKING CUISINE

AS YOU'VE LEARNED, there are many delicious foods that not only have a naturally low glycemic load but also act as sugar blockers, helping to slow down your body's absorption of starches. And as I've noted before, because starch is largely tasteless, when you replace it with other foods, you will actually be increasing the amount of flavor and texture in your diet. In fact, I bet you'll find that you're eating even better than you did before.

In this chapter you'll find more than 50 scrumptious recipes to help you incorporate these amazing sugar-blocking foods into your meals. In addition, there are some cooking techniques and eating strategies that can help you avoid blood sugar spikes.

● STARCH SUBSTITUTES

The easiest way to turn your high-glycemic meals into low-glycemic ones is, of course, by replacing the starchy foods in your meals with nonstarchy ones. Here are some ideas for common starches.

▶ **Pasta:** They don't call it spaghetti squash for nothing! Cut a spaghetti squash in half and microwave at full power for 10 minutes, or until a knife pierces easily into the flesh. Using a fork, scrape out the squash into a large bowl and separate into strands. Voilà—you have a great substitute for spaghetti or any other kind of noodle you might want to enjoy. Zucchini strands can also work. Or try shirataki noodles, a Japanese dish that's low in carbs. You can usually find them in the Asian section of supermarkets or in health food stores.

▶ **Potato and rice:** It's white and filling, and you can bake, roast, boil, or mash it. Surprise! This versatile vegetable is cauliflower, and as it turns out, it makes a very handy, nonstarchy substitute for potatoes. Try cauliflower in soups and stews, as a hearty side dish, and even in "potato" salads; you'll see just how similar it is. Plus, the taste of cauliflower, like that of potatoes, is mild enough that you can season it any way you like. Cauliflower can also stand in for rice, believe it or not; just shred it into small pieces and microwave in a couple of tablespoons of water for 5 to 6 minutes.

▶ **Bread:** Instead of making a sandwich for lunch, chop up your sandwich fillings and serve them over salad greens. Not only will you get more fiber that way, but you won't be left with a huge head of lettuce rotting in your fridge because you've used only a few leaves to garnish your sandwich! Or, if you really want a handheld meal, wrap your fillings in a large piece of lettuce instead. You can also use low-carb tortilla wraps to substitute for bread. Look at the numbers for total carbohydrate and fiber, and subtract the fiber from the carbs. If the difference is 13 grams or less per serving, the wrap won't raise your blood sugar as much as a slice of white bread would.

● BAKING WITH NONSTARCH FLOURS

As you know, most baked goods are full of starch; however, you can significantly lower the glycemic load of baked goods by using nonstarch flours. In this chapter, you'll find several recipes to help you learn how to bake with nonstarch flours. To create them, I enlisted the help of several expert recipe developers. In these recipes they used almond meal or coconut flour mixed with a small amount of whole grain pastry flour to get the best texture and taste.

▶ **Almond meal:** As with most nut flours, almond meal contains more oil than wheat flour, so you won't need as much butter as usual. You will, though, need more eggs to bind the dough; it's a little more crumbly than flour because of the lack of gluten. Egg whites will also help lighten the dough, which tends to be heavier than wheat flour. Also, because the

JANE WILCHAK

JANE WILCHAK LOVED TRYING OUT new sugar-blocking foods to keep the Sugar Blockers Diet fun and exciting. "Don't think of it as a diet—it's not a diet; it's an eating plan," she said. "It's a great program, and it's easy. It helped me step up my creativity."

Jane roasted cauliflower with sea salt, crushed black pepper, and oil for a sumptuous mashed potato substitute. She added chia seeds to ice cream for a sugar-blocking crunchy sweet treat (the extra fiber also helped her lactose-sensitive stomach cope with her dairy-heavy diet). "I fell in love with almond milk," she reported, "I use it with cereal and everything. Eating cereal with milk used to upset my stomach, but this doesn't."

Great flavor hasn't been the only benefit for Jane: "I feel great. My concentration is better, I'm more productive at work, and I'm exercising again." Even her 14-year-old son, Zack, who has type 1 diabetes, has noticed changes in his own measures. His after-meal sugar levels dropped from more than 200 down to the low 100s.

For Jane, one of the best things about meal planning has been that she never overeats anymore. Before starting the plan, she'd pick at the ingredients while cooking and at the leftovers while cleaning up. Now she eats nuts or a stick of cheese before dinner if she's hungry, and she stops eating when she feels full—but not overly full. "This way I'm able to get up after dinner, clear the table, and say, 'Let's go for a walk.'" In fact, after-dinner walks have been beneficial for both Jane and her husband, who use it as a chance to spend some quality time together at the end of each day.

"I've started to feel really good about myself," she added. "Things are fitting better and I've lost inches, which is a big deal for me. It keeps me motivated as I continue to see success and stay physically active."

Age: 44
Lost 6 pounds and
9" in 6 weeks

oil means that you have a larger amount of moisture in the dough, you will need longer baking times.

▶ **Coconut flour:** Like almond meal, coconut flour is denser and tends to clump more than wheat flour, so you'll need more eggs to bind and lighten the dough. And unlike almond meal, coconut flour can be a bit dry, so you may need more butter and/or some pureed fruit (such as applesauce) to add moisture.

● COOKING AL DENTE

As you learned in Chapter 4, there are a number of stops along the digestive path where you can help slow the breakdown of starches into sugars. One such stop actually occurs before you even put starchy foods in your mouth. Because larger particles of food are harder to break down, cooking your starches in a way that creates larger particles is a helpful sugar-blocking technique. When choosing pasta, for instance, favor larger pieces (such as lasagna) over smaller shapes (such as orzo). And cook your pasta so that it is firm, not soft. The common term for this is *al dente,* an Italian phrase meaning "to the bite" or "to the tooth." If you're not used to it, this may seem as though it's undercooked, but it is in fact perfectly cooked. Most pasta packages give cooking times for al dente; if not, simply cook for about 3 minutes less than the suggested time.

This approach to cooking can be applied not just to pasta but also to rice, beans, and vegetables. In general, the less you cook a food, the longer it takes for you to digest it—and the slower your blood sugar is to rise.

● SUGAR-BLOCKING RECIPES

Now, on to the recipes! I worked with *Prevention* magazine's recipe developers to create a mix of different recipes to help you put the Sugar Blockers Diet into action. Some don't contain any starches at all and have naturally low glycemic loads. Others use starch substitutes or mimics to help you get the flavor and the texture of your favorite starches without the sugar-shocking effect. A few do include pasta, bread, or other starches, but they're combined with sugar blockers both to limit the amount of starch you're consuming and to slow its breakdown. And even where we have included starches, you'll see that we've included just enough to satisfy your tastebuds instead of relying on them to contribute to the overall filling effect of the meal. For example, if you love crab casserole, serve yourself a large portion of the crab and only as much rice as you need to feel that you're eating a rice casserole. The same idea with pasta. Make less spaghetti, more meatballs.

You'll see that we also worked as many different sugar blockers into the recipes as possible, so you won't have to resort to gulping down a couple of tablespoons of vinegar to get the sugar-blocking effects you need. (Besides, as you've learned, you get the best results when you combine various types of sugar blockers.)

And because sugar blockers are most effective when eaten before a starch-containing meal, we've brought back the first course. And they're not all salads (although there are lots of fun new salad combinations, of course, since they're the easiest way to get a good mix of sugar blockers)! You'll see some fatty snacks that you can munch on 10 to 30 minutes before you start your meal, as well as elegant appetizers you'd be proud to serve guests.

For the most part, we kept the total of the glycemic loads of the ingredients in each dish below 100—the glycemic load of a slice of white bread. As you'll recall, excessive consumption of foods with glycemic loads higher than 100 has been associated with increased risk of obesity and diabetes, while generous intake of foods with glycemic loads lower than 100 have been associated with reduced risk. Where the combined glycemic loads of the ingredients rose higher than 100, we added sugar blockers, which, according to research, reduce the glycemic load by at least one-third. And we encourage you to add even more sugar blockers of your choice.

Designed to be quick and easy to make (and easy to store so you can save leftovers for another day), these recipes can be used for busy weeknight dinners. Snack on Greek Tomato Poppers while preparing Grilled Steak and Fauxtatoes, or serve the simple and tasty Cucumber and Vinegar Salad to take the edge off your family's hunger while you roast the eggplant for Pasta alla Norma. Not only will these simple appetizers, snacks, and salads serve as great sugar blockers, but they'll also help you slow down and enjoy your meal so that you don't overeat. Plus, they'll make any day feel like a special occasion.

RECIPE FINDER

SUGAR-BLOCKING **RECIPES**

BREAKFASTS

SCRAMBLED EGGS WITH PESTO AND RICOTTA

SURE TO BECOME a favorite, this low-glycemic dish uses ricotta to add creaminess to ordinary scrambled eggs, while the pesto lends pizzazz and richness. If you're really short on time, scramble the eggs in the microwave as described in Chapter 10.

Prep time: 5 minutes
Total time: 10 minutes
Makes 1 serving

3 large eggs
1 tablespoon grated Parmesan cheese
   Pinch of ground black pepper
2 tablespoons whole milk ricotta cheese
1 tablespoon pesto

1. Heat a medium nonstick skillet coated with cooking spray over medium heat.

2. In a small bowl, beat the eggs, Parmesan, and pepper. Pour into the skillet. Cook for 2 minutes, stirring, or until the eggs are softly scrambled but still moist and creamy.

3. Spoon small dollops of the ricotta over the eggs and drizzle with the pesto. Stir briefly to just swirl into the eggs.

Per serving: 381 calories ▸ 27 g protein ▸ 3 g carbohydrates ▸ 29 g total fat ▸ 11 g saturated fat ▸ 0 g fiber ▸ 460 mg sodium

EGGS RANCHEROS

BLAND AND BORING EGGS reach new heights with this flavor-packed quick-and-easy breakfast. To make ahead, double the recipe except for the eggs and cheese, reserving half of the tomato mixture. The next day, bring it to a simmer and cook the eggs as directed.

Prep time: 10 minutes
Total time: 20 minutes
Makes 2 servings

½ teaspoon olive oil
2 scallions, sliced
2 cups frozen loose-pack spinach
¼ teaspoon ground cumin
1 can (8 ounces) no-salt-added tomato sauce
½ cup medium salsa
¼ cup water
2 eggs
⅓ cup shredded reduced-fat Mexican cheese blend

1. Heat the oil in a small skillet over medium heat. Cook the scallions, spinach, and cumin, covered, for 5 minutes, or until the spinach is just tender.

2. Stir in the tomato sauce, salsa, and water. Bring to a simmer. Make 2 shallow indents for the eggs. Crack the eggs one at a time and drop into the indentations. Cover and simmer for 3 minutes, or until the yolks are just soft. Remove from the heat.

3. Sprinkle with the cheese, cover, and let stand for 1 minute, or until melted.

Per serving: 299 calories ▶ 19 g protein ▶ 27 g carbohydrates ▶ 10 g total fat ▶ 4 g saturated fat ▶ 5 g fiber ▶ 858 mg sodium

BROCCOLI AND CHEESE MINI FRITTATAS

MAKE THESE ON A WEEKEND, and quickly microwave for a last-minute breakfast. Or tuck a frittata in with your lunch for a satisfying midday snack. Store in an airtight container in the refrigerator for up to 5 days.

Prep time: 20 minutes
Total time: 40 minutes
Makes 5 servings

2   cups frozen chopped broccoli (loose-pack)
2   scallions, chopped
½   teaspoon dried tarragon, crumbled
3   large eggs
3   large egg whites
⅓   cup unsweetened almond milk or milk
2   tablespoons almond flour
⅛   teaspoon salt
¼   teaspoon freshly ground black pepper
½   cup shredded reduced-fat extra-sharp Cheddar cheese
⅓   cup grated Parmesan cheese

1. Preheat the oven to 350°F. Coat 10 cups of a muffin pan with cooking spray. Heat a small nonstick skillet coated with cooking spray over medium heat. Cook the broccoli and scallions for 4 minutes, stirring occasionally. Stir in the tarragon and remove from the heat. Set aside to cool.

2. In a large bowl, whisk together the eggs, egg whites, milk, almond flour, salt, and pepper until blended. Stir in the Cheddar, Parmesan, and the broccoli mixture. Place ¼ cup of the mixture into each prepared muffin cup.

3. Bake for 20 minutes, or until the frittatas are set in the center. To remove, run a narrow rubber spatula or knife around the edge of each muffin cup to loosen.

Per serving: 149 calories ▶ 13 g protein ▶ 5 g carbohydrates ▶ 9 g total fat ▶ 4 g saturated fat ▶ 2 g fiber ▶ 341 mg sodium

BREAKFAST PIZZA

EGGS AND BACON ATOP a tortilla makes for a hearty and delicious, protein-packed start to the day. Feel free to substitute full-fat mozzarella cheese if you can't find reduced-fat. Although using a low-carb tortilla keeps the glycemic load low, the full-fat cheese will increase the sugar-blocking effect.

Prep time: 5 minutes
Total time: 15 minutes
Makes 1 serving

1   low-carb tortilla (6"–8" diameter)
⅓   cup shredded reduced-fat mozzarella cheese
1   large egg
2   slices cooked low-sodium bacon, cut into 1" pieces
1   tablespoon grated Parmesan cheese
    Pinch of ground black pepper

1. Preheat the oven to 425°F.

2. Place the tortilla on a baking sheet. Sprinkle with the mozzarella. Crack the egg into the center. Sprinkle with the bacon, Parmesan, and pepper.

3. Bake for 8 minutes, or until the egg white is set and the yolk is still runny.

Per serving: 337 calories ▸ 27 g protein ▸ 9 g carbohydrates ▸ 23 g total fat ▸ 9 g saturated fat ▸ 4 g fiber ▸ 775 mg sodium

SALMON BRUSCHETTA

THIS CLASSIC COMBINATION is a sure winner for a weekend breakfast. The protein and fat in the cream cheese and salmon help block the blood sugar–raising effects of the bread. Change it up by substituting one of a variety of flavored cream cheeses.

Prep time: 5 minutes
Total time: 10 minutes
Makes 2 servings

2   slices whole grain seeded sourdough bread, toasted
¼   cup chive-onion cream cheese
2   ounces smoked wild salmon
½   cucumber, peeled and thinly sliced

Place the bread on a work surface and spread the cream cheese on 1 slice. Top with the salmon and cucumber and the remaining slice of bread. Cut in half to serve.

Per serving: 307 calories ▸ 23 g protein ▸ 22 g carbohydrates ▸ 14 g total fat ▸ 8 g saturated fat ▸ 2 g fiber ▸ 374 mg sodium

BERRY WRAP

TRY DIFFERENT VARIATIONS of this delicious filling to start your day. Opt for raspberry preserves, raspberries, and chopped almonds for a change of pace. Or try flaxseeds instead of the chia seeds. Other fruit, such as sliced peaches or bananas, can also work. The possibilities are limited only by your imagination!

Prep time: 10 minutes
Total time: 15 minutes
Makes 1 serving

1	large low-carb whole wheat tortilla (9″ diameter)
2	tablespoons Neufchâtel cream cheese
1	tablespoon reduced-sugar strawberry preserves
¼	cup part-skim ricotta cheese
½	cup strawberries, hulled and sliced
¼	cup blueberries
2	tablespoons chopped walnuts
1	teaspoon chia seeds

1. Set the tortilla on a work surface and spread the Neufchâtel up to ½″ from the edges.

2. Spread the preserves over the Neufchâtel.

3. Spoon the ricotta in a strip on the lower third of the tortilla, about 1″ from the edge.

4. Top the ricotta with the strawberries, blueberries, walnuts, and chia seeds. Starting at the filled end, roll up the tortilla. Cut in half.

Per serving: 429 calories ▸ 21 g protein ▸ 44 g carbohydrates ▸ 26 g total fat ▸ 8 g saturated fat ▸ 18 g fiber ▸ 475 mg sodium

STEEL-CUT OATS AND QUINOA CEREAL

BREAKFASTS

BECAUSE 1 SERVING of this recipe accounts for your daily limit of starch, try topping this tasty cereal with fiber-rich blueberries or raspberries and full-of-good-fats walnuts or almonds. You can also stir in a fiber supplement or pair it with eggs or another protein-packed side.

Prep time: 5 minutes
Total time: 30 minutes
Makes 6 servings

½	cup steel-cut oats
½	cup quinoa, rinsed and drained
2	tablespoons chia seeds
1	apple, cored and chopped
1	teaspoon ground cinnamon
⅛	teaspoon salt
1	cup unsweetened almond milk or milk
1¼	cups water
2-3	packets (.035 ounce each) stevia

In a medium saucepan, stir together the oats, quinoa, chia seeds, apple, cinnamon, salt, milk, and water. Bring to a simmer and cook, covered, for 25 minutes, or until the grains are just tender, stirring occasionally. Stir in the stevia to taste and serve hot.

Per serving: 146 calories ▶ 5 g protein ▶ 25 g carbohydrates ▶ 4 g total fat ▶ 5 g saturated fat ▶ 5 g fiber ▶ 82 mg sodium

GREEN BANANA–NUT BREAD

TRADITIONALLY, banana bread is made with overripe bananas specifically because of their high sugar content. As bananas ripen, an enzyme in them turns the soluble fiber to sugar. But you want the exact opposite: more soluble fiber and less sugar. By using green bananas instead of brown ones, you get the banana flavor without all the sugar. You'll see that we've also replaced some of the flour with almond meal and added protein powder and walnuts to help block some of the blood sugar–raising effects of the bread.

Prep time: 15 minutes
Total time: 1 hour + cooling time
Makes 12 slices

- ¾ cup whole grain pastry flour
- ½ cup almond meal
- ½ cup vanilla whey protein powder
- ½ cup Sucanat
- ¾ teaspoon baking soda
- ¼ teaspoon cinnamon
- ¼ teaspoon salt
- 3 dark-green bananas
- ½ cup plain yogurt
- 2 large eggs
- 6 tablespoons butter, melted
- 1 cup chopped walnuts, toasted

1. Preheat the oven to 325°F. Coat a 9" x 5" loaf pan with cooking spray.

2. In a large bowl, whisk together the flour, almond meal, whey protein, Sucanat, baking soda, cinnamon, and salt.

3. In a medium bowl, mash the bananas with a fork. Stir in the yogurt, eggs, and melted butter. Add to the flour mixture along with the walnuts, stirring until just blended.

4. Place in the baking pan. Bake for 1 hour, or until a toothpick inserted in the center comes out clean. Cool in the pan on a rack for 10 minutes. Remove from the pan and cool completely.

Per serving: 244 calories ▸ 8 g protein ▸ 22 g carbohydrates ▸ 15 g total fat ▸ 5 g saturated fat ▸ 3 g fiber ▸ 160 mg sodium

PBJ-QUINOA PANCAKES

BREAKFASTS

IN THIS NEW TWIST on an old classic, you'll find tender pancakes bursting with peanut flavor and delicious topped with grape jelly. But if you prefer a different jelly option, select your favorite—strawberry, raspberry, or even apricot. If you can't find white chia seeds, feel free to substitute black ones. And since 1 serving of this recipe accounts for your 1-serving limit of starch, I'd suggest that you enjoy it with a generous helping of eggs, ham, bacon, or another sugar-blocking protein.

Prep time: 10 minutes
Total time: 40 minutes
Makes 6 servings

- ½ cup quinoa, rinsed
- 1 cup water
- ½ cup whole wheat pastry flour
- ¼ cup white chia seeds
- ½ teaspoon baking powder
- ¼ teaspoon baking soda
- ¼ teaspoon salt
- 1 cup buttermilk
- ⅓ cup natural chunky peanut butter
- 2 large eggs
- ¼ cup grape spreadable fruit

1. In a small saucepan, combine the quinoa and water. Bring to a boil. Reduce the heat to low and simmer for 10 minutes, or until the quinoa is tender and the water is absorbed. Turn the quinoa out onto a plate and let cool.

2. In a large bowl, whisk together the flour, chia seeds, baking powder, baking soda, and salt. In a small bowl, whisk together the buttermilk and peanut butter. Whisk in the eggs. Add the buttermilk mixture and quinoa to the flour mixture and stir until just combined. Let stand for 5 minutes.

3. Heat a griddle or a large nonstick skillet coated with cooking spray over medium heat. Working in batches if necessary, drop the batter by ¼ cupfuls onto the pan. Cook for 2 minutes, or until bubbles start to form on top. Turn with a spatula, and cook for about 3 minutes, or until browned, reducing the heat if necessary.

4. Place 2 pancakes on a plate and spread each with 1 teaspoon spreadable fruit.

Per serving: 257 calories ▶ 10 g protein ▶ 30 g carbohydrates ▶ 13 g total fat ▶ 2 g saturated fat ▶ 7 g fiber ▶ 318 mg sodium

RASPBERRY-APPLE SMOOTHIE

HERE'S A DELICIOUS, high-fiber fruit drink that you can make for a quick breakfast or refreshing snack. Including the peel (along with psyllium powder) bumps up the fiber quotient to counteract the sugar-shocking effect of "liquefying" the ingredients.

Prep time: 5 minutes
Total time: 5 minutes
Makes 1 serving

½ cup frozen or fresh raspberries
½ apple, cored and coarsely chopped
¾ cup unsweetened almond milk or fat-free plain yogurt
1 tablespoon unsweetened soy protein powder (optional)
2 teaspoons ground psyllium powder
4 ice cubes

In a blender, combine the raspberries, apple, milk or yogurt, protein powder (if using), psyllium powder, and ice cubes. Blend until smooth.

Per serving: 191 calories ▶ 3 g protein ▶ 46 g carbohydrates ▶ 3 g total fat ▶ 0 g saturated fat ▶ 16 g fiber ▶ 146 mg sodium

SUGAR-BLOCKING **RECIPES**

LUNCHES

SMOKED TURKEY, APPLE, AND GRAPE SALAD

BOTTLED VINAIGRETTE makes meal preparation a breeze. When selecting a brand, read all labels to be certain that there is no added sugar or corn syrup. Or you can use our easy Herbed Vinaigrette (page 187) with this recipe instead.

Prep time: 20 minutes
Total time: 20 minutes
Makes 4 servings

3   tablespoons bottled Italian vinaigrette
1   tablespoon sour cream
1   tablespoon white wine vinegar
1   tablespoon chia seeds (optional)
2   cups chopped fat-free smoked turkey breast
1   large apple, chopped
¾   cup halved grapes
2   ribs celery, sliced
1   package (10 ounces) mixed salad greens

In a medium bowl, stir together the vinaigrette, sour cream, vinegar, and chia seeds. Let stand for 5 minutes. Add the turkey, apple, grapes, and celery. Toss until well blended. Serve over the mixed greens.

Per serving: 138 calories ▶ 8 g protein ▶ 20 g carbohydrates ▶ 4 g total fat ▶ 1 g saturated fat ▶ 4 g fiber ▶ 642 mg sodium

HAM AND SWISS SALAD

NOT ONLY DOES this high-fiber take on an American favorite serve as a filling lunch on its own, but you can also try it as a delicious sugar-blocking appetizer—and a nice change from the standard green salad—before any starchy meal.

Prep time: 15 minutes
Total time: 15 minutes
Makes 4 servings

2   tablespoons cider vinegar
1½ tablespoons olive oil
2   teaspoons Dijon mustard
¼   teaspoon salt
⅛   teaspoon ground black pepper
4   ounces deli sliced ham, cut into strips
4   ounces sliced Swiss cheese, cut into strips
1   pear, quartered, cored, and sliced
1   rib celery, cut into strips
½   red bell pepper, thinly sliced
½   cup walnuts, coarsely chopped
4   cups packed baby salad greens

1. In a large bowl, whisk together the vinegar, oil, mustard, salt, and black pepper. Add the ham, cheese, pear, celery, bell pepper, and walnuts. Toss well to combine.

2. Divide the salad greens among 4 plates. Top with the ham-and-cheese mixture.

Per serving: 324 calories ▶ 16 g protein ▶ 14 g carbohydrates ▶ 24 g total fat ▶ 7 g saturated fat ▶ 4 g fiber ▶ 628 mg sodium

LUNCHES

CLASSIC COBB SALAD

TURN THIS INTO A SUPER COBB SALAD by adding some thinly sliced radishes, celery, and a chopped hard-cooked egg. You can also add a deli meat, such as ham or roast beef, for more protein, if you prefer.

Prep time: 15 minutes
Total time: 15 minutes
Makes 2 servings

1	small head romaine lettuce, chopped (6 cups)
¼	English cucumber, chopped
½	cup grape tomatoes
½	cup thinly sliced red bell pepper
½	small avocado, diced
4	ounces sliced low-sodium deli turkey breast, cut into short strips
2	tablespoons crumbled blue cheese
3	tablespoons reduced-fat vinaigrette
1	teaspoon white wine vinegar

Divide the lettuce between 2 plates. Top with mounds of the cucumber, tomatoes, bell pepper, avocado, turkey, and blue cheese. Drizzle each salad with 1½ tablespoons vinaigrette and ½ teaspoon of the vinegar.

Per serving: 245 calories ▶ 18 g protein ▶ 18 g carbohydrates ▶ 14 g total fat ▶ 3 g saturated fat ▶ 7 g fiber ▶ 811 mg sodium

SPINACH AND EGG SALAD

A WARM BACON DRESSING tops baby spinach, crunchy croutons, onion, and mushrooms. Keep in mind that the croutons count toward your 1-serving starch limit, so you may opt to leave them out or add more nuts or seeds to get that satisfying crunch without the sugar-shocking effects.

Prep time: 15 minutes
Total time: 30 minutes
Makes 2 servings

LUNCHES

1   bag (5 ounces) baby spinach
4   slices bacon, cut crosswise into 1½" pieces
2   slices whole grain seeded sourdough bread, cut into ½" cubes
1   red onion, halved and sliced
1   box (8 ounces) sliced cremini mushrooms
3   tablespoons natural rice vinegar
1   teaspoon Dijon mustard
¼   teaspoon pepper
1   tablespoon chia seeds
2   hard-cooked eggs, peeled and halved

1. Place the spinach in a large bowl.

2. In a large skillet over medium heat, cook the bacon for 5 minutes, or until crisp. With a slotted spoon, remove to a paper towel–lined plate. Pour off and reserve the bacon drippings.

3. Return 2 teaspoons of the bacon drippings to the skillet and heat over medium-low heat. Add the bread cubes and cook for 5 minutes, stirring frequently, or until lightly browned and crisp. Remove the croutons to a plate.

4. Add the onion and mushrooms to the skillet and increase the heat to medium. Cook for 4 minutes, stirring, or until the onion softens slightly. Stir in the vinegar, mustard, and pepper. Pour the mixture over the spinach. Add the chia seeds and toss to coat. Divide between 2 plates. Top each plate with one-half of the bacon, croutons, and eggs.

Per serving: 514 calories ▸ 21 g protein ▸ 37 g carbohydrates ▸ 33 g total fat ▸ 10 g saturated fat ▸ 9 g fiber ▸ 805 mg sodium

SOMEWHAT POTATO-AND-EGG SALAD

CHUNKS OF CAULIFLOWER stand in for potatoes in this mock potato salad. Once it's dressed, you'll hardly notice the difference. Serve with thin wedges of tomato.

Prep time: 15 minutes
Total time: 1 hour 15 minutes
Makes 4 servings

- 4 cups frozen cauliflower florets
- 1 large rib celery, chopped
- 2 tablespoons white wine vinegar
- 2 scallions, chopped
- ¼ teaspoon dried dill
- ¼ cup 0% Greek yogurt
- 3 tablespoons mayonnaise
- 1 teaspoon Dijon mustard
- ⅛ teaspoon salt
- ⅛ teaspoon red-pepper sauce
- 2 hard-cooked eggs, chopped
- ½ head iceberg lettuce, cut into wedges

1. Bring a large saucepan of water to a boil over high heat. Cook the cauliflower for 2 minutes only. (The water will just start to come to a boil.) Drain well, cut into bite-size pieces, and place in a large bowl. Add the celery, vinegar, scallions, and dill. Toss to combine. Cover and chill for at least 1 hour.

2. Add the yogurt, mayonnaise, mustard, salt, and pepper sauce. Toss until well blended. Gently stir in the eggs until combined and serve with the lettuce wedges.

Per serving: 158 calories ▶ 9 g protein ▶ 17 g carbohydrates ▶ 7 g total fat ▶ 1 g saturated fat ▶ 5 g fiber ▶ 289 mg sodium

PASTA AND CHICKPEA SALAD

THE FIBER-RICH, LOW-GLYCEMIC VEGETABLES in this salad help counteract the sugar-shocking effects of the pasta. Also, be careful not to overcook the pasta, and choose larger shapes, both of which help slow down its digestion.

Prep time: 20 minutes
Total time: 25 minutes
Makes 4 servings

LUNCHES

4   ounces whole grain rotelle pasta
1   cup canned chickpeas, rinsed and drained
1   small zucchini, chopped
1   carrot, shredded
½   small seedless cucumber, chopped
1½ cups grape tomatoes
2   scallions, chopped
⅓   cup chopped parsley
¼   cup light balsamic vinaigrette
1   tablespoon white wine vinegar
¼   teaspoon salt
¼   teaspoon red-pepper sauce

1. Prepare the pasta according to package directions, cooking to al dente. Rinse under cold water and drain well.

2. In a large bowl, toss together the pasta, chickpeas, zucchini, carrot, cucumber, tomatoes, scallions, parsley, vinaigrette, vinegar, salt, and pepper sauce.

Per serving: 216 calories ▸ 9 g protein ▸ 43 g carbohydrates ▸ 2 g total fat ▸ 0 g saturated fat ▸ 6 g fiber ▸ 446 mg sodium

VEGGIE–HUMMUS PITA

HERE'S A GREAT LAST-MINUTE SANDWICH when time is of the essence. The vinegar and chia seeds, along with the fiber in the hummus (made from chickpeas), all help block the blood sugar–raising effects of the pita. Try a variety of hummus flavors such as red pepper, pesto, and garlic.

Prep time: 5 minutes
Total time: 5 minutes
Makes 1 serving

⅓ cup prepared hummus
2 teaspoons chia seeds
2 tablespoons chopped kalamata olives
2 teaspoons white wine vinegar
1 small whole wheat pita, halved
¼ small cucumber, thinly sliced
½ vine-ripe tomato, sliced
1 leaf romaine lettuce, sliced

1. In a small bowl, stir together the hummus, chia seeds, olives, and vinegar.

2. Spoon and spread the hummus in each pita half and stuff with the cucumber, tomato, and lettuce.

Per serving: 296 calories ▶ 11 g protein ▶ 36 g carbohydrates ▶ 14 g total fat ▶ 2 g saturated fat ▶ 12 g fiber ▶ 797 mg sodium

ROAST BEEF AND MANGO ROLL-UPS

PUTTING FRUIT in these sandwiches adds a sweetness that balances the salty flavor of the meat. If you want to make them even lower in glycemic load, omit the tortillas and just roll everything up in lettuce leaves.

Prep time: 10 minutes
Total time: 10 minutes
Makes 2 servings

LUNCHES

3	tablespoons mayonnaise
1/2	teaspoon curry powder
1/2	teaspoon grated lime zest
1/2	teaspoon lime juice
2	low-carb tortillas (8" diameter)
4	ounces deli sliced roast beef
2	leaves green leaf lettuce
1/2	cucumber, peeled, seeded, and cut into strips
1/2	mango, cut into strips

1. In a small bowl, stir together the mayonnaise, curry powder, lime zest, and lime juice.

2. Lay the tortillas on a work surface and spread with half of the mayonnaise mixture. Top with the roast beef and lettuce. Arrange the cucumber and mango strips on the bottom third of each tortilla and roll up. Cut in half.

Per serving: 306 calories ▸ 16 g protein ▸ 17 g carbohydrates ▸ 21 g total fat ▸ 3 g saturated fat ▸ 5 g fiber ▸ 641 mg sodium

SHRIMP SALAD WRAPS

IF YOU LIKE, make 1 sandwich and refrigerate the shrimp salad mixture for up to 1 day. Try these wraps with cooked flaked salmon instead of the shrimp. For even lower carbs, skip the tortilla and just eat the salad on its own or wrap the salad in lettuce leaves.

Prep time: 15 minutes
Total time: 15 minutes
Makes 2 servings

3   tablespoons 0% Greek yogurt
1½ tablespoons mayonnaise
1½ teaspoons chia seeds
1   tablespoon fresh lemon juice
⅛   teaspoon salt
6   ounces large shelled and deveined cooked shrimp
½   carrot, shredded
½   rib celery, chopped
¼   red bell pepper, chopped
2   leaves lettuce
2   low-carb tortillas (8" diameter)

1. In a medium bowl, combine the yogurt, mayonnaise, chia seeds, lemon juice, and salt. Let stand for 5 minutes. Add the shrimp, carrot, celery, and bell pepper until combined.

2. Place a lettuce leaf in the center of each tortilla. Top with the shrimp mixture, roll up, and secure with picks.

Per serving: 225 calories ▶ 29 g protein ▶ 16 g carbohydrates ▶ 8 g total fat ▶ 1 g saturated fat ▶ 7 g fiber ▶ 596 mg sodium

SAUSAGE PIZZAS

A FASTER OPTION than calling for takeout, these high-fiber pizzas make a delicious lunch or light supper. Serve with veggie sticks or a tossed salad for the perfect sugar-blocking meal. Or eat just a small slice for a hearty snack.

Prep time: 10 minutes
Total time: 20 minutes
Makes 2 servings

2 cups broccoli florets, coarsely chopped
2 tablespoons water
2 low-carb tortillas (6"–8" diameter)
¼ cup grated Parmesan cheese, divided
2 plum tomatoes, coarsely chopped
2 fully cooked chicken sausages, cut into ½" slices
½ cup shredded reduced-fat mozzarella cheese

1. Preheat the oven to 425°F. In a medium microwaveable bowl, combine the broccoli and water. Cover with vented plastic wrap and microwave on high power for 2 minutes, or until the broccoli is tender-crisp. Drain and pat dry with paper towels.

2. Place the tortillas on a large baking sheet and sprinkle each with 1 tablespoon of the Parmesan. Top with the broccoli and tomatoes. Arrange the sausage slices on top. Sprinkle with the mozzarella and the remaining 2 tablespoons Parmesan.

3. Bake for 10 minutes, or until hot and the cheese melts. Let stand for 3 minutes before cutting each pizza into 4 slices.

Per serving: 350 calories ▶ 34 g protein ▶ 20 g carbohydrates ▶ 18 g total fat ▶ 7 g saturated fat ▶ 10 g fiber ▶ 805 mg sodium

LUNCHES

FIRST–COURSE APPETIZERS AND SALADS

SPICY TOMATO COCKTAIL

TOMATOES ARE A FRUIT with a low glycemic load, so they're an exception to the "no fruit juice" rule. Plus, the vodka makes this cocktail a sugar blocker. Enjoy with a handful of nuts for maximum sugar blocking.

Prep time: 10 minutes
Total time: 10 minutes
Makes 2 servings

2 cups low-sodium tomato juice, chilled
2 teaspoons hot sauce, or to taste
¼ cup vodka
1 teaspoon prepared horseradish
1 teaspoon Worcestershire sauce
¼ teaspoon celery salt
2 small ribs celery with leaves
2 dill pickle spears
1 small carrot, halved lengthwise
2 strips red bell pepper
2 lime slices

In a 2-cup glass measuring cup, combine the tomato juice, hot sauce, vodka, horseradish, Worcestershire sauce, and salt, stirring until blended. Pour into 2 glasses and garnish with the celery, pickles, carrot, bell pepper, and lime slices.

Per serving: 139 calories ▸ 3 g protein ▸ 16 g carbohydrates ▸ 0 g total fat ▸ 0 g saturated fat ▸ 4 g fiber ▸ 763 mg sodium

FIRST-COURSE APPETIZERS AND SALADS

LAYERED BEAN DIP

BLACK SOYBEANS are a good source of fiber and protein and can be substituted for yellow ones in most recipes. Remember to stick to raw vegetables for dipping rather than tortilla chips, which have a very high glycemic load.

Prep time: 20 minutes
Total time: 20 minutes
Makes 6 servings

1 can (15 ounces) black soybeans, rinsed and drained
¾ cup salsa
1 avocado, chopped
½ teaspoon ground cumin
½ cup reduced-fat sour cream
1 cup shredded reduced-fat Cheddar cheese
1 cup finely shredded romaine lettuce
  Raw vegetables for dipping, such as carrots, bell peppers, and celery

1. Place the beans in a 9" pie plate and coarsely mash some of the beans with a potato masher.

2. Spoon the salsa over the beans, spreading evenly. Top with the avocado and sprinkle with the cumin. Spread the sour cream over the avocado and sprinkle with the cheese and lettuce. Serve with the vegetables.

Per serving: 193 calories ▶ 12 g protein ▶ 10 g carbohydrates ▶ 13 g total fat ▶ 5 g saturated fat ▶ 6 g fiber ▶ 335 mg sodium

CAJUN NUT MIX

NUTS ARE A PERFECT first-course appetizer to block sugar. Cajun seasoning, hot sauce, and Worcestershire sauce add zest to the nuts. For a milder nut mix, substitute thyme, Italian seasoning, or herbes de Provence.

Prep time: 10 minutes
Total time: 30 minutes
Makes 10 servings

---

2   tablespoons unsalted butter
2   teaspoons Worcestershire sauce
2   teaspoons hot-pepper sauce
¾   cup unsalted roasted peanuts
¾   cup walnuts
½   cup almonds
½   cup pecans
1   teaspoon Cajun seasoning

1. Preheat the oven to 325°F. Line a rimmed baking sheet with foil.

2. In a large saucepan, heat the butter, Worcestershire sauce, and hot sauce over low heat for 2 minutes, or until the butter melts, stirring occasionally. Remove from the heat and add the peanuts, walnuts, almonds, and pecans. Toss to coat well. Sprinkle with the Cajun seasoning and stir well until evenly coated. Place on the prepared baking sheet.

3. Bake for 20 minutes, stirring once, or until the nuts are lightly toasted and dry. Let cool completely on a rack before serving.

....

Per serving: 208 calories ▸ 6 g protein ▸ 6 g carbohydrates ▸ 20 g total fat ▸ 3 g saturated fat ▸ 3 g fiber ▸ 91 mg sodium

SAVORY OAT SCONES

THESE SCOTTISH-STYLE SCONES are chock-full of oats, with some modern twists. If you don't have pepper jack cheese on hand, use an equal amount of Cheddar or fontina, and add 2 teaspoons chopped pickled jalapeño peppers. Because 1 serving of this recipe accounts for your 1-serving limit of starch, spread a little butter on them before eating or have some nuts on the side.

Prep time: 15 minutes
Total time: 30 minutes
Makes 8 servings

2   cups quick-cooking oats, divided
½   cup whole wheat pastry flour
1½ teaspoons baking powder
2   tablespoons chia seeds
½   teaspoon salt
½   cup grated pepper jack cheese
¼   cup grated Parmesan cheese, divided
½   cup milk
1   large egg
2   tablespoons canola oil

1. Preheat the oven to 400°F. Line a baking sheet with parchment paper.

2. In a food processor, pulse 1 cup oats for 1 minute, or until a fine meal. Place in a large bowl. Add the flour, baking powder, chia seeds, salt, pepper jack, 3 tablespoons of the Parmesan, and the remaining 1 cup oats. Stir to combine.

3. Make a well in the center. Add the milk, egg, and oil in the center. Stir together until blended. Let the mixture stand for 3 minutes.

4. Divide the dough in half. Drop the dough in 2 mounds on the prepared baking sheet. Using floured hands, pat each half of the dough into a 5" circle. Cut each round into 8 wedges. Sprinkle each wedge with ½ tablespoon of the remaining Parmesan. Bake for 15 minutes, or until a pick inserted comes out clean.

Per serving: 217 calories ▸ 9 g protein ▸ 22 g carbohydrates ▸ 10 g total fat ▸ 3 g saturated fat ▸ 4 g fiber ▸ 385 mg sodium

CURRIED CRAB DIP

THIS DELICIOUS DISH combines several sugar blockers—protein from the crab, fat from the cream cheese, fiber from the celery and apple—into a single powerful appetizer that's suitable for entertaining as well as for your own pleasure.

Prep time: 15 minutes
Total time: 15 minutes
Makes 5 servings
(⅓ cup)

2 teaspoons olive oil
½ red onion, finely chopped
1 clove garlic, crushed through a press
½ teaspoon curry powder
3 ounces cream cheese, softened
½ cup sour cream
1 tablespoon fresh lemon juice
¼ teaspoon salt
¼ teaspoon ground black pepper
1 can (6 ounces) crabmeat, drained
Celery sticks and apple slices

1. Warm the oil in a small skillet over medium-low heat. Cook the onion for 5 minutes, stirring occasionally, or until soft. Stir in the garlic and curry powder. Set aside to cool slightly.

2. In a blender or a food processor, combine the cream cheese, sour cream, lemon juice, salt, and pepper until smooth. Add the crabmeat and the onion mixture. Pulse just until blended. Place in a serving bowl. Cover and refrigerate for at least 1 hour to allow the flavors to blend. Serve with the celery sticks and apple slices.

Per serving: 152 calories ▸ 9 g protein ▸ 3 g carbohydrates ▸ 12 g total fat ▸ 6 g saturated fat ▸ 0 g fiber ▸ 300 mg sodium

GREEK TOMATO POPPERS

CAMPARI TOMATOES are larger than cherry tomatoes but smaller than vine-ripe tomatoes and make quick work for an appetizer portion. A melon baller will help save time when you're scooping out the tomatoes. Substitute large cherry tomatoes if you can't find Campari tomatoes.

Prep time: 15 minutes
Total time: 15 minutes
Makes 4 servings

- 2 tablespoons finely chopped red onion
- 4 tablespoons red wine vinegar, divided
- 12 Campari tomatoes
- 1/3 cup chopped seedless cucumber
- 1/2 cup crumbled feta cheese
- 6 kalamata olives, chopped
- 2 teaspoons chopped fresh oregano
- 1 tablespoon olive oil

1. Place the onion in a small bowl. Add 2 tablespoons vinegar and let stand for 10 minutes. Drain.

2. Meanwhile, trim the tops of the tomatoes and scoop out the centers. Toss together the cucumber, feta, olives, oregano, oil, drained onions, and the remaining 2 tablespoons vinegar. Spoon into the hollowed tomatoes and serve.

Per serving: 124 calories ▶ 4 g protein ▶ 6 g carbohydrates ▶ 10 g total fat ▶ 4 g saturated fat ▶ 1 g fiber ▶ 455 mg sodium

CREAMY PESTO RICOTTA

THE PROTEIN FROM THE RICOTTA and nuts, and fat from the pesto, make this appetizer a perfect sugar blocker. Feel free to swap another vegetable, such as cucumber or carrot, for the zucchini.

Prep time: 10 minutes
Total time: 10 minutes
Makes 4 servings

---

³/₄ cup whole-milk ricotta cheese
2   tablespoons pesto
1   medium zucchini, cut into about twenty ¼"-thick slices
¼   cup chopped walnuts

In a small bowl, stir together the ricotta and pesto. Spread the mixture on the zucchini slices. Sprinkle with the walnuts.

Per serving: 168 calories ▸ 8 g protein ▸ 3 g carbohydrates ▸ 14 g total fat ▸ 5 g saturated fat ▸ 1 g fiber ▸ 99 mg sodium

CUCUMBER AND VINEGAR SALAD

THIS REFRESHING RECIPE is delicious served with sliced tomatoes and shreds of cheese. The cucumber slices can also make good substitutes for bread-and-butter pickles in sandwiches. The vinegar acts as the sugar blocker.

Prep time: 15 minutes
Total time: 15 minutes
+ chilling time
Makes 4 servings

3 large cucumbers, peeled and thinly sliced
1½ teaspoons salt
¼ cup white vinegar
¼ cup cider vinegar
1 tablespoon Sucanat
1 tablespoon fresh chives, chopped

1. In a colander, toss together the cucumbers and salt until well blended. Place the colander inside a large bowl and chill for 1 to 2 hours.

2. In a large bowl, whisk together the white vinegar, cider vinegar, and Sucanat and stir until completely dissolved. Add the rinsed cucumbers and chives. Toss to coat well.

3. Chill for 2 hours or overnight.

Per serving: 41 calories ▶ 1 g protein ▶ 8 g carbohydrates ▶ 0 g total fat ▶ 0 g saturated fat ▶ 1.5 g fiber ▶ 732 mg sodium

FIRST-COURSE APPETIZERS AND SALADS

SPICY BEAN SALAD

SERVE THIS TASTY SALAD in hollowed-out tomato halves for a fun presentation. By using the beans cold, you avoid overcooking them, so they retain more of their sugar-blocking fiber. The vinegar and other vegetables also add to the sugar-blocking power of this dish.

Prep time: 20 minutes
Total time: 20 minutes
+ chilling time
Makes 6 servings

- ¾ pound green beans, cut in 1" pieces
- ¾ cup tomato juice
- ⅓ cup cider vinegar
- 2 tablespoons canola oil
- 1 teaspoon salt-free seasoning
- 2 teaspoons smoky hot-pepper sauce
- ½ packet stevia
- ½ teaspoon salt
- 1 can (15 ounces) black soybeans, rinsed and drained
- 1 can (15 ounces) kidney beans, rinsed and drained
- 4 scallions, chopped
  Mixed salad greens, for serving (optional)

1. Place a steamer basket in a large saucepan with 3" water. Bring to a boil over high heat. Add the green beans, cover, and steam for 10 minutes, or until tender-crisp. Rinse under cold running water and drain well.

2. Meanwhile, in a large bowl, whisk together the tomato juice, vinegar, oil, seasoning, hot sauce, stevia, and salt until blended. Add the soybeans, kidney beans, scallions, and the drained green beans. Toss together until evenly coated. Cover and refrigerate for at least 4 hours or up to 2 days.

3. Serve over the salad greens, if desired.

Per serving: 157 calories ▶ 8 g protein ▶ 16 g carbohydrates ▶ 7 g total fat ▶ 1 g saturated fat ▶ 7 g fiber ▶ 338 mg sodium

WARM RED CABBAGE SALAD

HEATING THE CABBAGE gives this salad a complexity that's delicious with walnuts, blue cheese, and red wine vinegar, all excellent sugar blockers. And it makes a great appetizer for pork or poultry dishes.

Prep time: 20 minutes
Total time: 25 minutes
Makes 4 servings

- 2 tablespoons olive oil
- ½ large head red cabbage, shredded
- ¼ cup red wine vinegar
- ⅓ cup walnuts, chopped
- ¼ cup chopped fresh flat-leaf parsley leaves
- ¼ teaspoon salt
- ¼ teaspoon ground black pepper
- ⅓ cup crumbled blue cheese

1. In a large skillet, heat the oil over medium-high heat. Cook the cabbage and vinegar for 3 minutes, stirring constantly, or until the cabbage is hot but still crunchy.

2. Remove the skillet from the heat and stir in the walnuts, parsley, salt, and pepper. Sprinkle with the blue cheese.

Per serving: 201 calories ▶ 6 g protein ▶ 10 g carbohydrates ▶ 17 g total fat ▶ 4 g saturated fat ▶ 3 g fiber ▶ 334 mg sodium

SESAME-GINGER GREEN BEAN SALAD

TRY THIS SALAD AS A FIRST COURSE or serve with grilled chicken breasts for an easy summer meal. The water chestnuts add a satisfying crunch, but if you want to boost your sugar-blocking efforts, use unsalted peanuts instead.

Prep time: 20 minutes
Total time: 20 minutes
Makes 4 servings

1 pound green beans, cut into 2" pieces
½ small red onion, sliced
1 can (8 ounces) sliced water chestnuts, rinsed and drained
¼ cup bottled Asian sesame dressing
½ teaspoon grated fresh ginger
2 tablespoons rice or white wine vinegar
½ teaspoon Sriracha chili sauce

1. Place a steamer basket in a large saucepan with 3" water. Bring to a boil over high heat. Add the green beans, cover, and steam for 10 minutes, or until tender-crisp, adding the onion during the last 2 minutes. Rinse under cold running water and drain well. Place in a large bowl.

2. Add the water chestnuts, dressing, ginger, vinegar, and chili sauce. Toss to coat well.

Per serving: 124 calories ▶ 3 g protein ▶ 15 g carbohydrates ▶ 7 g total fat ▶ 1 g saturated fat ▶ 4 g fiber ▶ 173 mg sodium

ZUCCHINI SALAD

THIN STRIPS OF ZUCCHINI tossed with tomato make a colorful and lovely first-course salad. Top with chopped nuts or grated cheese for variety and added sugar-blocking effect.

Prep time: 20 minutes
Total time: 20 minutes
+ marinating time
Makes 4 servings

- 2 tablespoons white wine vinegar
- 1 tablespoon canola oil
- ¼ teaspoon salt
- ⅛ teaspoon ground black pepper
- 1 tomato, seeded and chopped
- 1 shallot, very thinly sliced
- 2 small zucchini
- ½ cup fresh basil leaves, torn
- 2 teaspoons psyllium husks

1. In a large bowl, whisk together the vinegar, oil, salt, and pepper. Add the tomato and shallot. Toss to coat well. Let stand for 5 minutes.

2. With a vegetable peeler, shave thin lengthwise strips of the zucchini into the dressing, stopping at the seeded portion. Add the basil and toss to combine.

3. Divide the salad among 4 plates and sprinkle with the psyllium.

Per serving: 76 calories ▸ 3 g protein ▸ 10 g carbohydrates ▸ 4 g total fat ▸ 0 g saturated fat ▸ 3 g fiber ▸ 157 mg sodium

FIRST-COURSE APPETIZERS AND SALADS

ORANGE–WALNUT VINAIGRETTE

VINEGAR AND OIL are sugar blockers in this delicious vinai-grette with a hint of orange. Add to the sugar-blocking effects by tossing the vinaigrette in a veggie-packed salad sprinkled with chopped walnuts or chia seeds.

Prep time: 5 minutes
Total time: 5 minutes
Makes 4 servings
(2 tablespoons per serving)

¼ cup apple cider vinegar
¼ cup walnut or olive oil
1   tablespoon grated orange peel
¼ teaspoon salt
¼ teaspoon pepper

In a small jar with a tight-fitting lid, combine the vinegar, oil, orange peel, salt, and pepper. Cover and shake well until emulsified. Store in the refrigerator.

Per serving: 123 calories ▶ 0 g protein ▶ 1 g carbohydrates ▶ 14 g total fat ▶ 1.5 g saturated fat ▶ 0 g fiber ▶ 148 mg sodium

FIRST-COURSE APPETIZERS AND SALADS

HERBED VINAIGRETTE

A GREAT SUGAR BLOCKER, this classic dressing is delicious on mixed greens, steamed asparagus, and steamed cauliflower. Change the flavor by adding minced shallot or garlic or any blend of herbs.

Prep time: 5 minutes
Total time: 5 minutes
Makes 5 servings
(2 tablespoons per serving)

⅓ cup olive oil
¼ cup red wine vinegar
2 tablespoons chopped fresh basil
1½ teaspoons chopped fresh thyme
1 tablespoon Dijon mustard
¼ teaspoon salt
⅛ teaspoon freshly ground black pepper

In a small jar with a tight-fitting lid, combine the oil, vinegar, basil, thyme, mustard, salt, and pepper. Cover and shake well until emulsified. Store in the refrigerator.

Per serving: 134 calories ▸ 0 g protein ▸ 1 g carbohydrates ▸ 15 g total fat ▸ 2.5 g saturated fat ▸ 0 g fiber ▸ 189 mg sodium

DINNERS

GRILLED STEAK

TRY THIS DISH WITH GRILLED FISH or chicken in place of the steak. Add some fresh mint or basil to the herb sauce if you have it on hand. A mini food processor works well for the herb sauce. Serve this dish with the Mashed Fauxtatoes (page 201) for a complete steak dinner.

Prep time: 10 minutes
Total time: 30 minutes
Makes 4 servings

1	flank steak (1 pound), trimmed
4	tablespoons sherry vinegar, divided
1	tablespoon salt-free grilling-blend seasoning
½	cup packed cilantro leaves and stems
2	scallions
2	cloves garlic
1	tablespoon olive oil
¼–1	teaspoon jalapeño pepper sauce or red-pepper sauce
½	teaspoon dried marjoram
¼	teaspoon salt
2	tablespoons water

1. Place the steak in a shallow pan. Brush both sides with 2 tablespoons sherry vinegar and sprinkle on the seasoning. Set aside.

2. In a blender or food processor, combine the cilantro, scallions, and garlic until finely chopped. Add the oil, pepper sauce, marjoram, salt, water, and the remaining 2 tablespoons of the sherry vinegar. Pulse together until combined.

3. Coat the grates of a grill or grill pan with oil or cooking spray. Preheat a grill or grill pan over medium-high heat. Cook the steak for 8 minutes, turning once, or until a thermometer inserted in the center registers 145°F for medium-rare/160°F for medium/165°F for well-done. Let stand for 10 minutes before slicing. Thinly slice the steak across the grain. Serve with the cilantro sauce.

Per serving: 236 calories ▸ 24 g protein ▸ 3 g carbohydrates ▸ 13 g total fat ▸ 4 g saturated fat ▸ 0 g fiber ▸ 305 mg sodium

DINNERS

BEEF AND MUSHROOM STEW
WITH CARROT AND TURNIP SALAD

THE SLOW COOKER makes preparing this stew a cinch. If you'll be out of the house for longer than 4 hours, cook this stew on low for 7 to 8 hours. Feel free to pair with other salads if you prefer.

Prep time: 20 minutes
Total time: 4½ hours
Makes 6 servings

Beef and Mushroom Stew

1½ pounds beef-stew meat, divided
1   onion, chopped
1   can (14.5 ounces) reduced-sodium beef broth
4   cloves garlic, minced
1   box (8 ounces) sliced cremini mushrooms
1   cup water
½   teaspoon dried thyme
½   teaspoon salt
¼   teaspoon pepper

Carrot and Turnip Salad

3   carrots, shredded
1   turnip, peeled and shredded
3   tablespoons chopped parsley
2   tablespoons red wine vinegar
2   teaspoons olive oil
¼   teaspoon salt
⅛   teaspoon pepper

1. *To make the stew:* Heat a large nonstick skillet coated with cooking spray over medium-high heat. Cook half of the beef, turning, for 5 minutes, or until browned. Place in a 5-quart slow cooker. Repeat with the remaining beef. Add the onion to the skillet and cook, stirring, for 1 minute. Add the broth and garlic, stirring to scrape up any brown bits, and place in the slow cooker. Add the mushrooms, water, and thyme. Cover and cook on high for 4 hours, or until the meat is tender. Stir in the salt and pepper.

2. *Meanwhile, to make the carrot and turnip salad:* In a medium bowl, combine the carrots, turnip, parsley, vinegar, oil, salt, and pepper. Chill until ready to serve.

Per serving: 224 calories ▶ 28 g protein ▶ 9 g carbohydrates ▶ 8 g total fat ▶ 3 g saturated fat ▶ 2 g fiber ▶ 540 mg sodium

DINNERS

BUFFALO CHILI

IF YOU LIKE, SERVE THIS CHILI with chopped fresh cilantro, lime wedges, and chopped pickled jalapeño peppers.

Prep time: 15 minutes
Total time: 1 hour 10 minutes
Makes 4 servings

1   pound ground buffalo or beef
1   onion, chopped
4   teaspoons chili powder
2   teaspoons ground cumin
1   teaspoon oregano
3   cloves garlic, chopped
1   large red bell pepper, chopped
1   large green bell pepper, chopped
1   can (14.5 ounces) diced tomatoes
1   can (8 ounces) no-salt-added tomato sauce
1   tablespoon white vinegar
1   large zucchini, chopped
1   can (15 ounces) kidney beans, rinsed and drained
½   cup 0% Greek yogurt

1. Heat a Dutch oven over medium heat. Cook the beef and onion for 8 minutes, stirring, or until no longer pink. Stir in the chili powder, cumin, oregano, and garlic. Cook for 1 minute.

2. Stir in the red and green bell peppers, tomatoes, tomato sauce, and vinegar. Bring to a simmer. Cover and simmer for 35 minutes, stirring occasionally.

3. Stir in the zucchini and beans. Cook, uncovered, for 20 minutes, or until flavored through and the zucchini is tender. Serve with a dollop of yogurt.

Per serving: 350 calories ▸ 34 g protein ▸ 32 g carbohydrates ▸ 9 g total fat ▸ 3 g saturated fat ▸ 9 g fiber ▸ 479 mg sodium

DINNERS

PORK CHILI VERDE

SERVED WITH warmed low-carb tortillas and a tomato salad, this chili makes a filling lunch or dinner. A small cup of the protein-packed dish is also a good appetizer for a starchy meal.

Prep time: 25 minutes
Total time: 35 minutes
Makes 4 servings

---

2   tablespoons olive oil
1   pound pork tenderloin, cut into ¾" chunks
1   small onion, chopped
2   small zucchini, halved lengthwise and sliced crosswise
1   cup salsa verde
¾   cup low-sodium chicken broth
1   teaspoon ground cumin
½   avocado, peeled, seeded, and chopped
1   cup fresh cilantro, coarsely chopped

1. Heat the oil in a large nonstick skillet over medium-high heat. Cook the pork and onion for 5 minutes, stirring occasionally, or until lightly browned. Add the zucchini, salsa, broth, and cumin. Bring to a boil. Reduce the heat to medium and simmer for 5 minutes, or until the pork is cooked through and the zucchini is tender-crisp.

2. Divide among 4 bowls and sprinkle with the avocado and cilantro.

....

Per serving: 276 calories ▸ 26 g protein ▸ 9 g carbohydrates ▸ 15 g total fat ▸ 3 g saturated fat ▸ 4 g fiber ▸ 375 mg sodium

DINNERS

CHICKEN CACCIATORE

HERE, SPAGHETTI SQUASH serves as the perfect starch mimic for the classic Italian dinner. Topped with chicken in a flavorful and fiber-packed sauce, the squash is so delicious you'll never miss the pasta.

Prep time: 15 minutes
Total time: 35 minutes
Makes 4 servings

1   spaghetti squash (about 2½ pounds), halved crosswise and seeds removed
½   teaspoon salt, divided
1   teaspoon olive oil
1   onion, chopped
1   green bell pepper, chopped
1   package (10 ounces) mushrooms, quartered
⅓   cup dry red wine
¼   teaspoon crushed red-pepper flakes
1¼   pounds boneless, skinless chicken breast, cut into ½" pieces
1½   cups no-sugar-added light tomato-and-basil pasta sauce

1. Place the spaghetti squash cut side down on a large plate. Microwave at full power for 10 minutes, or until a knife pierces easily into the flesh. Using a fork, scrape out the squash into a large bowl and separate into strands. Toss with ¼ teaspoon salt.

2. Meanwhile, in a large nonstick skillet, heat the oil over medium-high heat. Cook the onion for 4 minutes, stirring occasionally. Add the bell pepper, mushrooms, wine, pepper flakes, and the remaining ¼ teaspoon salt. Cook for 6 minutes, stirring occasionally, or until the liquid is almost evaporated and the vegetables are just tender.

3. Stir in the chicken and pasta sauce. Bring to a simmer and cook for 6 minutes, or until the chicken is no longer pink. Place the spaghetti squash on dinner plates and spoon the cacciatore on top.

Per serving: 333 calories ▶ 36 g protein ▶ 30 g carbohydrates ▶ 7 g total fat ▶ 1 g saturated fat ▶ 7 g fiber ▶ 775 mg sodium

DINNERS

HERB-GARLIC CHICKEN

WITH THE GREEN BEANS and salad greens adding fiber and the chicken providing protein, this hearty sugar-blocking dish is also cooked in wine and topped with almonds (additional sugar blockers). It's ideal for dinner parties and everyday meals as well.

Prep time: 20 minutes
Total time: 30 minutes
Makes 4 servings

- ³⁄₄ pound green beans, trimmed
- 4 boneless, skinless chicken breast halves
- 1 teaspoon herb-garlic seasoning blend
- 2 teaspoons olive oil
- 2 large shallots, halved and thinly sliced
- ½ cup red wine
- ½ cup reduced-sodium chicken broth
- 2 tablespoons cold butter
- 1 tablespoon Dijon mustard
- 1 tablespoon red wine vinegar
- ¼ teaspoon salt
- 4 cups baby salad greens
- 2 tablespoons almonds, toasted and chopped

1. Bring 1" water to a boil in a large saucepan. Add the green beans and cook for 3 minutes. Drain and set aside.

2. Place the chicken between 2 sheets of plastic wrap and pound to ³⁄₄" thickness. Sprinkle both sides of the chicken with the seasoning blend.

3. In a large nonstick skillet, heat the oil over medium-high heat. Cook the chicken for 5 minutes, turning once, or until browned and cooked through. Transfer the chicken to a plate.

4. Reduce the heat to medium and cook the shallots for 2 minutes, stirring, or until slightly softened. Add the wine and broth and simmer for 5 minutes, or until reduced to 1 cup. Add the butter, mustard, vinegar, and salt. Cook for 2 minutes, stirring, or until the sauce thickens slightly and is reduced to ³⁄₄ cup. Return the chicken to the skillet and cook for 1 minute to heat through.

5. Place the chicken on 4 plates and top with the salad greens and the reserved green beans. Drizzle with the sauce and sprinkle with the almonds.

Per serving: 325 calories ▶ 30 g protein ▶ 17 g carbohydrates ▶ 14 g total fat ▶ 5 g saturated fat ▶ 4 g fiber ▶ 513 mg sodium

CRISPY PROSCIUTTO–CRUSTED CHICKEN

A COMPANY-WORTHY DISH that's simple enough to prepare on a weeknight. Start with a mixed green salad, and then serve the chicken with roasted or steamed broccoli for extra fiber.

Prep time: 15 minutes
Total time: 30 minutes
Makes 4 servings

4   boneless, skinless chicken breast halves
4   slices prosciutto or serrano ham
2   tablespoons whole grain pastry flour
1   tablespoon extra-virgin olive oil
1½ tablespoons butter, divided
4   large shallots, chopped
¾   cup dry white wine
¾   cup (3 ounces) shredded Italian fontina cheese
2   tablespoons capers in brine
2   tablespoons chopped fresh parsley
¼   teaspoon salt

1. Place the chicken between sheets of plastic wrap. Using a mallet or a heavy skillet, pound to ½" thickness. Place 1 slice prosciutto or serrano ham on the top side of each breast and press to adhere. Dip both sides of the chicken in the flour, shaking off the excess.

2. In a large nonstick skillet over medium-high heat, heat the oil and ½ tablespoon butter. Cook the chicken, ham side down, in the skillet for 8 minutes, turning once, or until no longer pink and the juices run clear. Remove to a plate and set aside.

3. Add the shallots and wine to the skillet. Cook for 4 minutes, or until reduced to about ¼ cup, scraping up any bits on the bottom of the pan. Return the chicken to the skillet and sprinkle with the cheese.

4. Reduce the heat to medium-low, cover, and cook for 3 minutes, or until the cheese melts. Place the chicken on a platter. Stir in the capers, parsley, salt, and the remaining 1 tablespoon butter, until blended. Spoon over the chicken and serve.

DINNERS

Per serving: 418 calories ▸ 38 g protein ▸ 19 g carbohydrates ▸ 19 g total fat ▸ 8 g saturated fat ▸ 1 g fiber ▸ 951 mg sodium

SAUSAGE AND PEPPERS

FOR THIS CLASSIC DISH, crush the fennel seeds in a mortar and pestle, or wrap in foil and crush on a cutting board with a heavy skillet. If you'd like to have this sandwich-style, hollow out a hot dog bun to reduce the glycemic load or try wrapping the sausage and peppers in a low-carb wrap.

Prep time: 10 minutes
Total time: 45 minutes
Makes 4 servings

1¼ cups water, divided
1 package (16 ounces) hot or sweet Italian turkey sausages
1 tablespoon olive oil
1 large onion, halved and sliced
3 large red bell peppers, sliced
2 large green bell peppers, sliced
2 cloves garlic, chopped
1¼ teaspoons Italian seasoning
2 tablespoons balsamic vinegar
¾ teaspoon fennel seeds, crushed
¼ teaspoon salt

1. In a large skillet over medium heat, bring 1 cup water to a boil. Add the sausages and cook, covered, for 6 minutes, turning once. Pour off the water.

2. Add the oil and cook for 6 minutes, or until browned and cooked through. Remove the sausages to a plate and set aside. When cool enough to handle, slice thickly on the diagonal.

3. Add the onion to the skillet and cook for 5 minutes, or until softened. Increase the heat to medium-high. Stir in the red and green bell peppers, garlic, seasoning, and the remaining ¼ cup water. Cover and cook for 10 minutes, or until the peppers are tender-crisp.

4. Stir in the vinegar, fennel seeds, salt, sausages, and any accumulated juices. Cook for 5 minutes, stirring occasionally, or until the sausages are heated and the vegetables are flavored through.

Per serving: 286 calories ▶ 24 g protein ▶ 17 g carbohydrates ▶ 13 g total fat ▶ 3 g saturated fat ▶ 5 g fiber ▶ 829 mg sodium

DINNERS

MEDITERRANEAN BAKED COD

VEGETABLES, THE MAIN COURSE, and the sauce all bake together in this one-pan meal—it's delicious and easy and has a low glycemic load. Because 1 serving of this recipe contributes to your daily limit of starch, I'd suggest having a hearty salad before eating the cod. Or try substituting cauliflower "rice."

Prep time: 15 minutes
Total time: 30 minutes
Makes 4 servings

- 2 zucchini, thinly sliced
- 2 yellow squash, thinly sliced
- 1 red onion, thinly sliced
- 1 teaspoon olive oil
- ¾ teaspoon salt-free lemon-pepper seasoning
- ¼ teaspoon salt
- 1 can (14.5 ounces) petite-diced tomatoes, drained
- 3 tablespoons chopped green olives
- ¼ cup chopped parsley
- 4 cod fillets (5 ounces each)
- ¼ cup slivered fresh basil
- 1½ cups cooked brown rice
  Lemon wedges, for serving

1. Preheat the oven to 425°F. In a 13" x 9" baking dish, combine the zucchini, squash, onion, oil, seasoning, and salt. Bake for 10 minutes, stirring once.

2. Meanwhile, in a medium bowl, combine the tomatoes, olives, and parsley. Arrange the cod fillets on top of the zucchini. Spoon the tomato mixture over the fillets.

3. Bake for 12 minutes, or until the fish flakes. Sprinkle with the basil and serve with the rice and lemon wedges.

Per serving: 289 calories ▶ 30 g protein ▶ 32 g carbohydrates ▶ 4 g total fat ▶ 1 g saturated fat ▶ 5 g fiber ▶ 579 mg sodium

DINNERS

FISH TACOS

USING LOW-CARB TORTILLAS keeps the glycemic load low, but if you prefer more traditional corn tortillas with these tacos, be sure to have a fatty or a fiber-rich snack beforehand for extra sugar blocking. The high-fiber coleslaw tossed with vinegar, and the fish and cheese, also make good sugar blockers for the starch in the corn tortillas.

Prep time: 20 minutes
Total time: 30 minutes
Makes 4 servings

1 pound tilapia fillets, cut into $\frac{3}{4}$" chunks
$1\frac{1}{2}$ teaspoons chili powder
2 tablespoons canola oil, divided
1 teaspoon ground cumin
$\frac{1}{4}$ teaspoon salt, divided
3 cups coleslaw mix
2 tablespoons red wine vinegar
4 warmed low-carb tortillas (6" diameter)
1 tomato, chopped
1 cup fresh cilantro leaves
$\frac{1}{2}$ cup shredded reduced-fat pepper jack cheese

1. Preheat the oven to 425°F. Coat a baking sheet with sides with cooking spray.

2. In a large bowl, combine the tilapia, chili powder, 1 tablespoon oil, cumin, and $\frac{1}{8}$ teaspoon salt. Toss to coat well. Place on the baking sheet. Bake for 10 minutes, or until the fish is opaque.

3. Meanwhile, in a medium bowl, combine the coleslaw mix, vinegar, the remaining 1 tablespoon oil, and the remaining $\frac{1}{8}$ teaspoon salt. Toss to mix.

4. To serve, spoon the fish into the tortillas and serve with the coleslaw mix, tomato, cilantro, and cheese.

Per serving: 328 calories ▶ 32 g protein ▶ 22 g carbohydrates ▶ 14 g total fat ▶ 2 g saturated fat ▶ 4 g fiber ▶ 678 mg sodium

DINNERS

PASTA ALLA NORMA

ROASTING THE EGGPLANT not only saves prep time but also intensifies the flavor. If you like the texture of the eggplant peel, pare it in alternating 1"-wide strips down the length of the eggplant. The fat in the oil and cheese, the fiber in the eggplant, and the vinegar in the capers all help block the blood sugar–raising effect of the pasta in this dish. Be sure to have a sugar-blocking first course prior to this meal.

Prep time: 25 minutes
Total time: 50 minutes
Makes 4 servings

2   unpeeled cloves garlic
2   teaspoons olive oil
1   eggplant (about 1¼ pounds), cut into ½" cubes
1   onion, chopped
¼   teaspoon salt
6   ounces whole grain pasta
1½ cups no-sugar-added jarred light pasta sauce
1   tablespoon capers
¼   teaspoon red-pepper flakes
¼   cup fresh chopped basil or parsley
½   cup part-skim ricotta cheese

1. Preheat the oven to 425°F. Wrap the garlic in a 6" square of foil. Coat a baking sheet with sides with cooking spray. Drizzle with the oil.

2. Place the eggplant and onion on the baking sheet. Sprinkle with the salt. Bake the eggplant and garlic for 30 minutes, or until tender, stirring once.

3. Meanwhile, prepare the pasta according to package directions, cooking to al dente. Remove the garlic from the foil, peel, and finely chop.

4. Heat the sauce, capers, pepper flakes, and the garlic in the pasta pot for 2 minutes, or until hot. Add the eggplant mixture, pasta, and basil or parsley and toss until well blended. Divide among 4 pasta bowls and top each with 2 tablespoons ricotta.

Per serving: 335 calories ▶ 13 g protein ▶ 50 g carbohydrates ▶ 11 g total fat ▶ 2 g saturated fat ▶ 12 g fiber ▶ 518 mg sodium

DINNERS

PENNE WITH BROCCOLI RABE AND BEANS

FRESH BROCCOLI RABE is less intense in flavor than frozen and best used for this dish. To be certain, try tasting a piece of the stem for bitterness. If it's too strong, blanch the rabe for 2 minutes in boiling water and drain well. Have a fiber-rich salad and a fatty snack before eating the pasta.

Prep time: 35 minutes
Total time: 35 minutes
Makes 4 servings

2	tablespoons olive oil
1	large onion, halved and sliced
2	red bell peppers, cut into short, thin strips
2	cloves garlic, thinly sliced
½	teaspoon red-pepper flakes
1	bunch (1¼ pounds) broccoli rabe, cut into 1" pieces
¾	cup low-sodium vegetable broth
6	ounces whole grain penne
1	cup cannellini beans, rinsed and drained
2	tablespoons white balsamic vinegar
½	teaspoon salt
½	cup grated Romano cheese, divided

1. Heat the oil in a large skillet over medium heat. Cook the onion for 4 minutes, or until softened. Add the bell peppers, garlic, and pepper flakes. Cook for 2 minutes, stirring occasionally.

2. Stir in the broccoli rabe and broth. Bring to a simmer and cook for 8 minutes, or until the vegetables are softened.

3. Meanwhile, prepare the pasta according to package directions, cooking to al dente. Drain and return to the pasta pot. Add the beans, vinegar, salt, ¼ cup cheese, and the rabe mixture. Toss together and serve with the remaining ¼ cup cheese.

Per serving: 423 calories ▸ 21 g protein ▸ 52 g carbohydrates ▸ 13 g total fat ▸ 4 g saturated fat ▸ 11 g fiber ▸ 674 mg sodium

MASHED FAUXTATOES

MASHED CAULIFLOWER makes the perfect starch mimic for high-glycemic load potatoes. Adding sour cream gives a delicious richness to the mash.

Prep time: 10 minutes
Total time: 40 minutes
Makes 4 servings

1 head (about 1¼ pounds) cauliflower, cut into florets
3 scallions, chopped
⅓ cup reduced-fat sour cream
¼ teaspoon salt

1. Place a steamer basket in a large saucepan with 3" water. Bring to a boil over high heat. Add the cauliflower, cover, and steam for 25 minutes, or until very tender, adding the scallions during the last 10 minutes. Carefully remove the steamer basket. Drain the saucepan well.

2. Return the cauliflower and scallions to the saucepan and cook over medium heat for 3 minutes, stirring occasionally or until dry. Remove from the heat. Add the sour cream and salt. Mash with a potato masher or hand blender.

Per serving: 76 calories ▶ 4 g protein ▶ 9 g carbohydrates ▶ 3 g total fat ▶ 2 g saturated fat ▶ 3 g fiber ▶ 349 mg sodium

DINNERS

SUGAR-BLOCKING **RECIPES**

SNACKS/DESSERTS

STRAWBERRIES WITH BITTERSWEET-CHOCOLATE SAUCE

THIS SIMPLE DESSERT is so delicious, you can serve it after a quick dinner or a special meal. Thanks to its good fats and fiber, it can also work as a sugar-blocking snack before a starchy meal.

Prep time: 15 minutes
Total time: 20 minutes
Makes 6 servings

½   cup heavy cream
4   ounces bittersweet 70% chocolate
2   tablespoons chopped crystallized ginger
1½ pounds strawberries, hulled and halved
3   tablespoons almonds, toasted and chopped

1. Place the cream in a small microwaveable bowl. Microwave on high power for 1 to 2 minutes, or until hot. Add the chocolate and let stand for 1 minute. Whisk until the chocolate melts and the sauce is smooth. Stir in the ginger.

2. Divide the strawberries among 4 dessert plates. Spoon the chocolate sauce over the strawberries and sprinkle with the almonds.

Per serving: 250 calories ▸ 4 g protein ▸ 24 g carbohydrates ▸ 18 g total fat ▸ 9 g saturated fat ▸ 5 g fiber ▸ 13 mg sodium

MIXED-BERRY SHORTCAKES

ALMOND FLOUR AND HIGH-FIBER BERRIES block the starches in the whole grain pastry flour in this classic summer treat. You can substitute full-fat Greek yogurt for the 0% fat version if you prefer.

Prep time: 25 minutes
Total time: 40 minutes
Makes 8 servings

Biscuits
- ¾ cup whole grain pastry flour
- ¾ cup almond meal/flour
- 1 tablespoon Sucanat
- 1½ teaspoons baking powder
- ¼ teaspoon baking soda
- ¼ teaspoon salt
- ½ cup buttermilk
- 2 tablespoons canola oil
- 1 large egg white
- 1 tablespoon fresh lemon juice
- 1 teaspoon grated lemon zest

Filling
- 2 cups strawberries, sliced
- 1 cup blueberries
- ½ cup raspberries
- 2 tablespoons Sucanat, divided
- 1 cup 0% plain Greek yogurt

1. *To make the biscuits:* Preheat the oven to 400°F. Coat a baking sheet with cooking spray. In a large bowl, combine the pastry flour, almond meal, Sucanat, baking powder, baking soda, and salt.

2. In a medium bowl, whisk together the buttermilk, oil, egg white, lemon juice, and lemon zest until well blended. Add to the flour mixture and stir just until the dough comes together.

3. Turn the dough out onto a lightly floured surface. Knead 10 times. Pat to an 8" x 4" rectangle. Cut into 8 square biscuits. Using a wide spatula, lift each biscuit onto the baking sheet. Bake for 14 minutes, or until golden brown. Remove to a rack to cool.

4. *To make the filling:* In a medium bowl, combine the strawberries, blueberries, raspberries, and 1 tablespoon Sucanat. Let stand for 15 minutes, stirring occasionally.

5. In a small bowl, combine the yogurt and the remaining 1 tablespoon Sucanat. Let stand for 15 minutes, stirring occasionally.

6. Split the biscuits crosswise in half. Place a biscuit bottom on each of 8 dessert plates. Top each with the berry mixture and a spoonful of the yogurt. Cover with the biscuit tops.

Per serving: 194 calories ▶ 8 g protein ▶ 22 g carbohydrates ▶ 9 g total fat ▶ 1 g saturated fat ▶ 4 g fiber ▶ 241 mg sodium

SNACKS/DESSERTS

PLUMS POACHED IN SPICED WINE

SERVE THESE with a dollop of light sour cream for a classy dessert. Or enjoy a half portion of the fruit with $\frac{1}{3}$ cup Greek yogurt for a zesty, sugar-blocking snack before a starchy meal.

Prep time: 10 minutes
Total time: 15 minutes
Makes 4 servings

- $\frac{3}{4}$ cup dry red wine
- 2 tablespoons all-fruit cherry jam
- 1 small star anise (or 2 whole cloves)
- $\frac{1}{4}$ teaspoon ground cinnamon
- $\frac{1}{4}$ cup water
- 4 plums, pitted and cut into 8 wedges

1. In a small saucepan, combine the wine, jam, star anise, cinnamon, and water. Bring to a simmer, stirring, until the jam is dissolved. Add the plums and simmer for 5 minutes, or just until tender when pierced with a knife.

2. Remove the star anise and discard. Set aside to cool completely. (It can be made up to 2 days in advance. Keep refrigerated.)

Per serving: 88 calories ▶ 1 g protein ▶ 14 g carbohydrates ▶ 0 g total fat ▶ 0 g saturated fat ▶ 1 g fiber ▶ 2 mg sodium

SNACKS/DESSERTS

NUTTY BROWNIES

HERE'S A MOUTHWATERING TREAT that's sure to satisfy your chocolate cravings. The walnuts, almond flour, eggs, and butter block the sugar-spiking impact of the flour. Just limit yourself to 1 serving, please!

Prep time: 15 minutes
Total time: 35 minutes
Makes 16 brownies

¾ cup Sucanat
¼ cup butter, melted
2 large eggs
1 teaspoon vanilla extract
⅓ cup unsweetened cocoa powder
¼ cup whole grain pastry flour
¼ cup almond or coconut flour
¼ teaspoon baking powder
⅛ teaspoon salt
⅓ cup bittersweet chocolate chips
½ cup chopped walnuts, divided

1. Preheat the oven to 350°F. Coat an 8" x 8" baking pan with cooking spray.

2. In a large bowl, whisk together the Sucanat, butter, eggs, and vanilla until well blended. Stir in the cocoa powder, pastry flour, almond or coconut flour, baking powder, and salt.

3. Stir in all but 2 tablespoons of the walnuts and the chocolate chips. Place in the prepared pan. Sprinkle with the remaining 2 tablespoons walnuts.

4. Bake for 20 minutes, or until a toothpick inserted in the center comes out with moist crumbs. Cool completely in the pan on a rack.

Per brownie: 138 calories ▶ 3 g protein ▶ 14 g carbohydrates ▶ 9 g total fat ▶ 3 g saturated fat ▶ 1 g fiber ▶ 41 mg sodium

CHOCOLATE FLOURLESS CAKE

ALMOND FLOUR AND EGGS create a delicious, dense, rich cake while keeping the glycemic load relatively low. You certainly won't feel as if you're on a diet as you enjoy this decadent dessert!

Prep time: 20 minutes
Total time: 45 minutes
Makes 8 servings

---

3 ounces unsweetened chocolate, chopped
2 tablespoons butter
⅓ cup reduced-fat sour cream
2 egg yolks
1 tablespoon vanilla extract
1 teaspoon espresso powder
¾ cup + 2 tablespoons Sucanat
½ cup almond flour
¼ teaspoon salt
5 egg whites, at room temperature

1. Preheat the oven to 350°F. Line an 8" springform pan with parchment paper and coat the bottom and sides with cooking spray.

2. Place the chocolate and butter in a large microwaveable bowl. Microwave for 2 minutes, stirring every 45 seconds, or until the chocolate is melted and smooth. Set aside for 10 minutes.

3. Whisk in the sour cream, egg yolks, vanilla, and espresso powder until blended. Add ¾ cup Sucanat, the almond flour, and salt. Whisk together until well blended.

4. In a large bowl, with an electric mixer on high speed, beat the egg whites until foamy. Gradually add the remaining 2 tablespoons Sucanat, beating, until stiff peaks form.

5. Add one-quarter of the beaten whites into the chocolate mixture and beat on low just until combined. Fold in the remaining whites in 2 additions, mixing just until combined. Spoon into the pan.

6. Bake for 25 to 40 minutes, or until the cake is dry on the top and a wooden pick inserted in the center comes out with a few moist crumbs. Cool on a rack until warm. (The cake will deflate.) Loosen the edges of the cake with a knife and remove the pan sides. Cut into wedges to serve.

Per serving: 262 calories ▶ 7 g protein ▶ 26 g carbohydrates ▶ 14 g total fat ▶ 7 g saturated fat ▶ 1 g fiber ▶ 132 mg sodium

SNACKS/DESSERTS

CARROT CAKE CUPCAKES

NUTS, CARROTS, COCONUT FLOUR, cinnamon, and cream cheese all work as sugar blockers in these tasty treats. One cupcake makes a perfect little dessert.

Prep time: 30 minutes
Total time: 55 minutes
+ cooling time
Makes 12 cupcakes

1   cup whole grain pastry flour
1/3 cup coconut flour
1 1/2 teaspoons ground cinnamon
1   teaspoon baking powder
1   teaspoon baking soda
1/4 teaspoon salt
2   large eggs
3/4 cup + 1 teaspoon Sucanat
1/2 cup unsweetened applesauce

1/3 cup canola oil
1/4 teaspoon + 4 drops vanilla-flavor
     stevia extract (liquid stevia)
1/2 pound carrots, shredded (2 cups)
1/2 cup chopped pecans, divided
1/4 cup golden raisins or dried
     apricots, chopped
4   ounces cream cheese, softened
2   teaspoons milk

1. Preheat the oven to 350°F. Line a 12-cup muffin pan with paper liners.

2. In a medium bowl, combine the pastry flour, coconut flour, cinnamon, baking powder, baking soda, and salt.

3. In a large bowl, combine the eggs, 3/4 cup Sucanat, the applesauce, oil, and 1/4 teaspoon stevia. Using an electric mixer on low speed, beat until well blended. Let stand for 10 minutes. Add the flour mixture and beat on medium speed for 1 minute, or until smooth. Stir in the carrots, 1/4 cup pecans, and the raisins or apricots. Divide the batter among the muffin cups.

4. Bake for 25 minutes, or until a toothpick inserted in the center of the cupcakes comes out clean. Cool in the pan on a rack for 5 minutes. Remove from the pan and cool completely on a rack.

5. In a medium bowl, with an electric mixer on low speed, beat the cream cheese, milk, the remaining 1 teaspoon Sucanat, and the remaining 4 drops stevia until fluffy. Frost the cupcakes and sprinkle with the remaining 1/4 cup pecans.

Per cupcake: 246 calories ▶ 4 g protein ▶ 27 g carbohydrates ▶ 14 g total fat ▶ 3 g saturated fat ▶ 4 g fiber ▶ 257 mg sodium

MOCHA GRANITA

THIS IS CHOCOLATEY ENOUGH to satisfy the deepest of cravings. For a creamier version, scrape the frozen granita into a food processor and pulse for 10 to 15 seconds, or until smooth. Serve with a dollop of whipped cream for a rich sugar-blocking effect, but you can also eat this after a meal of meat and vegetables.

Prep time: 10 minutes
Total time: 5 hours
Makes 6 servings

- ½ cup Sucanat
- ¼ cup unsweetened cocoa powder
- ⅛ teaspoon salt
- 1 cup water
- 3 ounces unsweetened chocolate, chopped
- 2 cups strong brewed coffee
- ¼ cup spoonable stevia (about 16 packets)
- 1 tablespoon vanilla extract
- ⅛ teaspoon ground nutmeg

1. In a large saucepan, combine the Sucanat, cocoa powder, salt, and water and bring to a boil. Reduce the heat to medium and cook for 2 minutes, stirring constantly, or until the Sucanat is dissolved. Remove the saucepan from the heat and stir in the chocolate, whisking until melted and smooth. Stir in the coffee, stevia, vanilla, and nutmeg until blended.

2. Pour the mixture into a 9" × 9" baking pan. Cover tightly with foil and freeze for 3 hours, or until frozen along the edges. With a fork, scrape the ice from the edges toward the center. Repeat 4 times at 30-minute intervals, or until the granita is semifirm.

3. To serve, use a fork to scrape across the surface of the granita, transferring the ice shards to 6 dishes or wineglasses. Serve at once.

Per serving: 153 calories ▸ 3 g protein ▸ 23 g carbohydrates ▸ 8 g fat ▸ 5 g saturated fat ▸ 4 g fiber ▸ 64 mg sodium

SNACKS/DESSERTS

10

NEGOTIATING
A CARB-FILLED
WORLD

NOW YOU KNOW HOW to eat the Sugar Blockers Diet way. You know what foods you need to cut back on: starches and sugar-containing beverages. You know how to combine sugar blockers like vegetables, nuts, chicken, cheese, and vinegar into scrumptious snacks, salads, and appetizers that will help you avoid dangerous sugar shocks and make it easy to lose weight. You have an arsenal of simple cooking techniques and recipes that you can use to battle the excess insulin that is making you fat.

But I know you're busy and don't always have time to cook. Some days you barely have a minute to eat! And what do you do when you're at a business lunch or a friend's potluck dinner, or rushing through the airport, and it seems the only things to eat are chips and cookies?

In this chapter, I'll share with you a few tricks I've learned through my years of sugar blocking that will help you navigate the carb-filled waters of the modern diet.

● SUGAR-BLOCKING TRICKS

One good thing about starch is that it's easy to see. You don't need to memorize the list of starch-containing foods in Chapter 8 to know what to avoid. However, if there is any doubt about how much a particular snack might raise your blood sugar, you can draw some useful conclusions by looking at the ingredient list on the package label.

Use Ingredient Lists to Estimate Glycemic Load

Your rule of thumb: Remember the unlucky number 13. That's how many grams of carbohydrates are in a slice of white bread. If something contains fewer than 13 grams of carbohydrates, you know that it can't raise your blood sugar higher than a slice of white bread would. A slice of white bread has a glycemic load of 100, so the glycemic load of the food in question must be less than 100. For example, if the package ingredient list says that a square of chocolate contains 4 grams of carbohydrates, under the worst-case scenario—if you absorbed it as fast as white bread—it couldn't raise your blood sugar as much as a slice of white bread would, simply because it doesn't contain enough carbs.

You can be more exact than that. Because the chocolate square has less than half the carbs of a slice of white bread, you can conclude that its glycemic load is less than half that of a slice of white bread—less than 50. That means you could eat two squares and not exceed a glycemic load of 100. You still don't know how fast the carbs would be absorbed—the other ingredients in the chocolate (fats in the chocolate, for instance, or nuts) could act as sugar blockers and reduce the glycemic load further. All you can say is that even if its carbs were absorbed as fast as those in white bread, the glycemic load would still be less than 100.

Build a Starch Pile

You don't need to be good at math to put this technique to work, but you do need to know how to use a knife and fork. If your mother scolded you for picking at your food and praised you for being a member of the "Clean Plate Club," it's time to disobey Mom and join the "Messy Plate Club." Just because someone puts a bunch of starch on your plate doesn't mean you have to eat it all. Really. The cook might be miffed if you don't eat the entrée, but nobody's feelings are going to be hurt if you leave some potatoes on your plate. In fact, it's good manners to leave a little food uneaten; it lets your host know that you've had enough to eat.

One good thing about starch (perhaps the only good thing) is that it's easy to separate from other food. A good trick is to build a starch pile on one side of your plate and delay eating from it until you've finished most of your meal. This gives the other food a chance to satisfy your hunger before you start eating from the starch pile. You may find that seeing all that tasteless paste in a big pile reduces your appetite for it. Just remember that you're looking at a pile of future sugar. When you finish your meal, you can congratulate yourself: You've staved off a sugar shock.

Even if you do help yourself to some of that starch at the end of your meal, at least you won't be eating it on an empty stomach. Whatever sugar blockers you had with your meal will help blunt the starch's effects on your blood sugar.

Take a Walk

If you slip up and eat some starch, there's one last way you can reduce its effects on your blood sugar: Take a walk. A brisk 20-minute walk immediately after eating will open up channels in your muscle cells and allow them to take up glucose independent of how much exercise you have done that day.

Consider Acarbose

As discussed in Chapter 4, acarbose is a pharmaceutical starch blocker that reduces after-meal blood sugar levels, promotes weight loss, and helps prevent diabetes. A natural substance produced by soil bacteria, acarbose is among the safest pills you can take. It doesn't even enter the bloodstream. Serious side effects are practically unheard of.

Because acarbose was developed to treat diabetes, it is available by prescription only (see Chapter 13). However, your doctor can prescribe it "off-label" to help you manage your weight and forestall diabetes.

If you take acarbose immediately before eating a starch-containing meal, it will reduce the impending blood sugar surge by as much as 40 percent. You don't have to take it regularly. In fact, it makes no sense to take acarbose with meals that contain little or no starch. Some patients carry a few tablets in their wallet or purse in case they're caught in situations in which starch can't be avoided.

● A DAY OF REAL-WORLD EATING

Armed with the strategies you've learned in this book, you're ready to take on our carb-filled world. First let's look at a typical day meal by meal—breakfast, lunch, and dinner.

A Typical American Breakfast

What is a typical American breakfast? Forty years ago, you might have said bacon, eggs, and a glass of milk. However, we eat differently now. After we were told we shouldn't eat so much cholesterol, we started eating more baked goods, breakfast cereals, and orange juice. Now we're also fatter and more diabetic. Could there be a correlation?

Tufts University researchers had a group of subjects eat eggs for breakfast and compared their eating behavior for the rest of the day with that of another group that ingested the same number of calories in the form of instant oatmeal. The group that ate the oatmeal consumed an astonishing *81 percent* more calories in the last half of the day than did the ones who ate the eggs for breakfast. Other researchers have found that high–glycemic load breakfasts cause people to eat more and gain more weight than low–glycemic load ones.

If you're going to give yourself a sugar shock, breakfast is the worst time of day to do it. Your body is more prone to sugar shocks early in the day than later. When you start your day with a sugar shock, your blood sugar tends to fluctuate for the rest of the day.

We Americans like lots of variety when it comes to dinner, but at breakfast time we seem to be short on imagination. We're content with the same old things—eggs, cereal, or baked goods like toast, bagels, and doughnuts. Of those choices, eggs are the only one that won't cause your blood sugar to shoot up. Unless you start eating a wider assortment of foods—meat, fish, cheese, vegetables—for breakfast, as people in other countries do, you're stuck with eggs.

Today, Americans are eating 23 percent fewer eggs than we did before 1970. One reason is we're in too much of a hurry to cook them, so instead we gulp down some orange juice, grab a bagel and a cup of coffee, and we're out the door. If time is a problem for you in the morning, I have a suggestion: Do as they do in Paris; microwave an omelet. Trust me, it's good. Here's how you do it.

Break a couple of eggs in a bowl, add a glop of milk, and whip it up as if you're going to make a regular omelet, then stick it in the microwave. Cook it for 3 minutes 30 seconds at 40 percent power, then take a peek. If you see liquid, nuke it another 20 seconds on full power. Take it out, plop a little butter on it, add salt and pepper, and enjoy. The good thing about microwaving eggs is that it's precise. You can cook them perfectly. You can add other ingredients, such as onions, cheese, tomatoes, and meat. However, you'll probably find that when the eggs are cooked to perfection, as you can do with a microwave, you enjoy them without all of the other goodies.

If you must have toast with your egg, stick to one piece and make sure that you don't eat the toast before the egg. As discussed in Chapter 7, the protein in the egg will improve the efficiency of your insulin response and reduce the blood surge from the toast.

If you're really missing your cereal, try an all-bran cereal. As I mentioned in Chapter 6, wheat bran is the best source of insoluble fiber in the American diet and has the lowest glycemic load of common American cereals. A lot of folks don't like the flavor of bran, though; they say it tastes like cardboard. This is probably because bran cereal is short on oil and protein. A good fix? Add a few tablespoons of chia seeds or a handful of chopped walnuts; both are sugar blockers and contain plenty of protein and healthy unsaturated oils. That can make bran cereal into a much heartier and tastier breakfast. You can also add berries or a spoonful or two of another cereal to make it tastier.

Also, as you learned in Chapter 9, you can still have the occasional muffin or pancake as long as you make it with nut flours to block the effects of whatever starch it contains and add other sugar blockers like berries and nuts.

A Typical American Lunch

Generally, Americans enjoy a wider variety of foods for lunch than we do breakfast. However, the quintessentially American midday meal is the sandwich. One reason it's popular is that you don't need a knife, fork, plate, chair, and table to eat it. You can sit on a stump, pick up your sandwich with your hands, and eat it. Or even eat it while you're walking and talking, in true American multitasking fashion.

When it comes to your blood sugar, the problem with a sandwich, of course, is the bread. The glycemic load of a couple American-size slices of bread (42 grams per slice) is approximately 300. That's your starch allotment for the entire day.

So how do you get the convenience of a sandwich and the taste you're used to without shooting up your blood sugar? Learn to make a "wrap"— a sandwich made with a tortilla. An 8-inch wheat tortilla has a glycemic load of 80, which is less than a single slice of bread. The glycemic loads of low-carb tortillas are even less. "I discovered the low-carb wraps and love them," said tester Jane Wilchak.

Wraps are easy to make. Just put all of the ingredients you would normally include in a sandwich on top of a tortilla, roll it up into a tube, and fold one end so that the filling doesn't fall out when you pick it up. If you're packing your lunch, wrapping it in plastic wrap will help hold it together.

Or, as you learned in Chapter 9, turn your sandwich fillings into toppings for an entrée-size salad, with the works—meat, cheese, nuts, olives, avocados, mushrooms, tomatoes, and any kind of dressing you like. It's a shame to put all of those sugar blockers to waste, so have a little bread if you want. Just make sure you eat it *after,* not before, you eat the salad.

A Typical American Dinner

What could be more American than meat and potatoes? A typical American dinner frequently includes a small salad, some type of meat (usually beef or chicken), vegetables on the side, and a starch (potato, pasta, or rice), with a beverage and something sweet for dessert. Most of these foods are fine; the problem is the starch—let's say it's a baked potato. Here's how a savvy eater would handle it.

First, have a fatty snack—a handful of nuts, a piece of cheese, or a couple of pork rinds—10 to 30 minutes before you eat your meal. The fat will pass into your small intestine, which will send signals to your stomach telling it to empty more slowly. This helps keep the meal you're about to eat from being digested too quickly. It's okay to have a beverage with your fatty snack, but refrain from drinking liquids during your meal. This will prevent the food in your stomach from liquefying too quickly, which speeds digestion.

Next, eat your salad. It will provide soluble fiber to soak up glucose and slow its absorption into your bloodstream. Consider adding nuts, olive oil, cheese, chunks of vegetables, or a vinegar-based dressing—all of which inhibit starch absorption—to your salad. You can also use vinegar as a condiment and sprinkle it on other foods. It substitutes well for salt.

Eat as much of your vegetable as you can, which will add to the salad's fiber. By now you should be approaching 10 grams of fiber.

Cut your potato in half, then alternate bites of potato with bites of meat. The protein in the meat causes insulin to be secreted more promptly, which improves its efficiency and lessens the total amount you have to produce to handle the starch.

You can have anything you want for dessert, as long as it's small enough for the fingers of one hand to wrap around it. A few squares of chocolate, some chocolate-covered nuts, or a half-dozen jelly beans should suffice. Dessert is for satisfying your sweet tooth, not for filling up. If you're still hungry, eat more vegetables or meat.

● DINING OUT

Whether you eat at a hamburger joint or a chain restaurant or go in for ethnic cuisine, starch will be on the menu because it's filling and, above all, cheap. No worries. Sugar blockers will help you deal with virtually any dining situation. As tester Renee Marchisotto said: "You just take a look at things and step back and see what's available. You can even go to fast-food chains and stay within the plan."

A Hamburger Joint

How can you live in America without eating the occasional hamburger? Here's how to keep America's most popular fast-food item from giving you glucose shock.

Actually, most of the ingredients in a deluxe burger with all the trimmings—cheese, mayo, mustard, pickles—are fine. They won't raise your blood sugar at all; in fact, some of them serve as sugar blockers. The problem, of course, is the bun. It has a glycemic load of 213—about the same as two slices of bread.

If you're making a burger at home, you can treat it like other sandwiches and turn it into a wrap. Cook up a thick piece of hamburger, cut it into inch-wide strips, and wrap each strip in a low-carb tortilla with the usual trimmings. Another way to do it is to put a patty between several leaves of iceberg lettuce, using the lettuce as a bun.

If you're eating out, the object is simple: Get rid of as much of the bun as possible. You can order a hamburger without the bun and eat it with a

MICHELLE NEWHARD

MICHELLE NEWHARD and her husband, Scott, are always on the go—and with both of them working full-time and raising two boys, they are always looking for more hours in the day. After 10 years of marriage, the couple realized that, between the demands of work and home, they hadn't been taking enough care of themselves, and they decided to join the Sugar Blockers Diet as a way to refocus on their health and stop the slow calorie creep before it set them back even further. As extra motivation, Michelle wanted to shed a few pounds as a present to herself. "I want to celebrate my 40th in a big way this year, and conquering this weight loss goal of mine will definitely help!" she said. "Plus, both Scott and I need to be strong and healthy into our sixties and seventies so we can spend time with grandkids!"

While Michelle and Scott were working on resetting their metabolism to keep up with current kids and future grandkids, Michelle's father, Bruce, saw a similar opportunity and joined the program with them, making it a real family affair! And everyone saw benefits: Scott lost more than 12 pounds, and Bruce shed significant points from his triglyceride level.

"When we were stressed, it worked. When we were relaxed, it worked. For big birthdays it worked. Takeout, comfort

Age: 39
Lost 4½ pounds
and 6" in 6 weeks

knife and fork. Cooks these days are used to serving burgers this way. You may be surprised how delicious a good piece of hamburger is with all the trimmings and without all that bread getting in the way.

If you like the taste of hamburger bun, notice that the top bun is about twice as big as the bottom one. If you remove it, you reduce the

food, every situation . . . it worked," Michelle said, adding that it felt good to be able to fit everything in—watching what she and Scott ate, what the kids ate, making time for exercise. "I didn't think it would ever work."

And they all found something to eat on the Sugar Blockers Diet "menu." Michelle said her two young boys were very into the cheese sticks and Slim Jims—sugar-blocking snacks that weren't very hard on the family's food budget. And as a result, the boys' energy level changed, too. "Before, they would fill up on starches and be hungry 5 minutes later, then another 10 minutes later," she said. But by following this plan, Michelle discovered changes even in her children—they're now "focusing more at school."

She put her own newfound energy to good use, too, finding it easier to concentrate at work and still make time to work out afterward. "I signed up for two 5-Ks, and this was a really great way to get me motivated," she said, adding that the exercise has helped her take time to release the stress of being a working mom and also helped her sleep better at night. "My back pain went away, too. I had low-energy days like everyone else, but I never wanted to quit. That never happened before. That was the best feeling—not having to force myself to follow through."

Three generations of Michelle and Scott's family have benefited from lessons learned in sugar blocking, and they plan to stick with it!

"I found that hummus is a great party food to use as a dip with raw vegetables."

glycemic load to approximately 70. Thus, another way to have a burger is to remove the top bun and eat it as an open-faced sandwich or with a knife and fork.

Of course, all of those methods require you to fiddle around with your burger, when all you want to do is pick it up and eat it. It's *fast* food, right? Well, here's the hassle-free, ultrafast way to do it: Pick up the burger, and just before you take a bite, break off a bite-size hunk of the top bun exactly where you're about to take a bite and put it in your starch pile. You may find its flavor better because you're not diluting the flavor with so much bread. It shouldn't raise your blood sugar much at all.

Instead of ordering fries, have a salad before your burger to further reduce your after-meal blood sugar.

A Full-Service Restaurant

Considering the choices you have in a full-service restaurant, you should have no trouble crafting a good low–glycemic load meal. However, no matter how upscale a restaurant is, the management is going to try to get you to fill up on starch so you won't want to eat so much of the expensive stuff. That's why they bring you free bread before your meal.

Remember the Sugar Blockers Diet rule number one: Never eat starch on an empty stomach. Resist eating more than the equivalent of a half slice of bread before your meal. However, if you want a bite or two, you can use it as a vehicle for a before-meal fatty snack. Break off a piece, slather it with about a teaspoon of butter, and eat it. Do it twice, and you've changed a sugar shocker into a sugar blocker.

One good thing about most full-service restaurants today is that they offer a wide variety of salads, some of which are quite hearty, containing meat, cheese, nuts, and vegetables. The more of these ingredients a salad has, the better it blocks sugar.

The entrées typically include a starch. However, ask if you can have extra vegetables instead. Waiters are used to that these days.

Desserts are usually much larger than you need just to satisfy your sweet tooth. Instead, wait until you get home to have a few bites of something sweet. If you have no shame, you can bring your own chocolate to the restaurant and sneak a few nibbles as you linger over coffee. They won't kick you out before you pay your bill. If you must have dessert in the restaurant, stick to fruit-based, creamy, or nutty desserts rather than cakes or brownies.

A Mexican Restaurant

You'll encounter danger at every turn here. Chips, tacos, and tortillas made with corn flour raise blood sugar even more than similar foods made with wheat flour. A lot of dishes at Mexican restaurants are served with rice or refried beans, which raise your blood sugar more than freshly cooked ones.

If you skip the rice and beans, however, it's possible to enjoy a good Mexican meal without triggering a glucose shock—as long as you employ sugar-blocking techniques. Guacamole is an excellent choice for a before-meal fatty snack. It contains healthy unsaturated oils and protein, and won't raise blood sugar at all. But beware of the tortilla chips. It takes only six measly chips to raise your blood sugar as much as a slice of white bread.

Here's how to eat chips and guacamole without giving yourself a glucose shock. Use your chip as a spoon. Dip the chip into the guacamole and spoon it into your mouth without eating the chip, or just eat a little to add crunch. If you are sharing the guacamole with friends, you may not want to stick the tortilla chip back into the guacamole dish after it's been in your mouth. In that case, put a slug of guacamole on your plate and spoon it from that. And stick to just three chips.

A good choice for an entrée is a fajita—strips of grilled meat served with sautéed peppers, onions, guacamole, sour cream, salsa, and tomato, none of which will raise your blood sugar. However, fajitas are served with tortillas. Mixing the ingredients together with your knife and fork and eating them without the tortilla is delicious. People often wrap the ingredients in the tortilla and eat it like a wrap. If you want to eat it that way, have just one tortilla. Tear off about a quarter of the tortilla, and wrap it around a couple forkfuls of ingredients and eat it with your fingers.

An Italian Restaurant

For many Americans, Italian cuisine is synonymous with pasta—a high–glycemic load culprit. An entrée-size serving of spaghetti (approximately 2 cups) has a glycemic load of more than 400. Eating that much pasta has the same effect on your blood sugar and insulin levels as choking down two hamburger buns all at once. If you're going to have pasta, you need to take measures to soften the sugar shock.

It's almost as if the Italians knew that you needed sugar blockers with your pasta. Italian restaurants serve great fatty appetizers—antipasti, which literally means "before pasta." Traditional favorite antipasti include caprese, which is sliced mozzarella cheese, tomatoes, and basil drenched in olive oil; carpaccio, thin slices of tenderloin dressed in oil and topped with capers and Parmesan cheese; prosciutto, thin slices of uncooked ham; and marinated olives. Bread is dipped in olive oil and vinegar—both primo sugar blockers. You can also get a salad with plenty of sugar-blocking ingredients, and the balsamic vinegar they use has a high acetic acid content, the active sugar-blocking ingredient of vinegar. Have a glass of wine, another good sugar blocker.

Now take a look at your pasta choices. You'll notice that many Italian restaurants serve pasta as *primi*, or first courses. In other words, it's not your entrée! These are smaller portions but can still be enough to raise your blood sugar if you're not careful. Order a pasta dish that has plenty of other ingredients—meat, seafood, olives, olive oil, and vegetables, all sugar blockers. As you eat, separate some of the pasta from the other ingredients, and put it in your starch pile. If the dish is, say, half pasta and half other ingredients, and if you push aside a third of the pasta, your sugar blockers should bring the glycemic load down to the point of giving you a mild blood sugar surge instead of a sugar shock.

Then you can enjoy your *secondi* course—usually a meat or fish dish—without worrying about your blood sugar. To finish your meal in style, skip the tiramisu and the cannoli, and instead enjoy a cup of espresso, followed by a nice walk.

Pizza

Pizza is a cinch to handle. Whether you go for a classic like pepperoni or want to get more adventurous with buffalo chicken or artichokes and anchovies, most toppings are low carb. The problem is the crust. The glycemic load of the crust in one slice is 70 percent of that of a slice of white bread. Have three slices, and you're pushing your glycemic load limit for the entire day.

Here's the trick. Just don't eat that big hunk of dough at the base of the triangle. Put it in your starch pile. If you do that, you reduce the glycemic load by about two-thirds. That means you can eat three slices without exceeding the glycemic load of a slice of white bread.

Chinese and Japanese Restaurants

Chinese and Japanese restaurants have delightful meat, poultry, chicken, fish, and vegetable dishes that do not contain starch. However, many do include rice, which, as you know, is solid starch. The glutinous rice used for sushi is especially bad. Noodles, including rice noodles, also have high glycemic loads.

Although Asians have been eating rice for thousands of years, they didn't consume as much of it as they do today. Separating the starchy cores from the husks was labor-intensive. It was considered a delicacy to be enjoyed in small amounts. Only since the advent of rice-polishing machines in the 1920s has rice become the staple it is today. Now Asia has some of the fastest-rising obesity and diabetes rates in the world.

Try this: Instead of using meat and vegetables to flavor the rice, think in reverse. Use a few spoonfuls of rice or noodles to mellow out the flavors of the meat and vegetables. One-half cup or so consumed with meat and vegetables shouldn't spike your blood sugar.

On the Road

If you're traveling by car, you can usually eat when you want and at whatever kind of restaurant you want. Air travel is another story. You're trapped in an airplane for hours at a time with nothing to eat but pretzels, or waiting in an airport with a limited selection of restaurants. You may arrive at your destination at odd hours and can't always choose where you will be when hunger hits. You're often compelled to eat things that you would normally try to avoid, such as starchy snacks and fast food.

Here's a suggestion: Bring along some nuts. They're among the healthiest foods you can eat, they're easy to carry, you can enjoy them anytime, and they'll do an excellent job of curbing your appetite. They will put you back in control of your hunger when you're traveling.

Also, if you're planning to eat at restaurants and you tend to crave a bite or two of something sweet after meals, consider packing some chocolate or another starch-free sweet snack. Rather than eating the huge desserts that restaurants usually offer, you can have your own, more appropriate-size dessert later.

And bring your walking shoes. I once talked to an airline pilot who gained weight after he stopped working. When he was flying and had layovers in cities away from home—often several times a week—he brought his walking shoes and explored the cities on foot. That kept his weight down until he retired.

● LOOK AT THE BRIGHT SIDE

It's hard to be happy about being overweight or having insulin resistance, especially if it ends up causing type 2 diabetes. But now you know that you don't lack self-discipline or have some sort of psychological problem. Your lifestyle is no different from other people's. The problem is that you have a hormonal imbalance: Your body makes too much insulin when you eat the large amounts of refined carbohydrates typical of the modern diet.

To turn your health around, you don't have to plumb the depths of your willpower and deprive yourself of satisfying amounts of good food. You just need to cut out a few starchy culprits. Considering that starch is largely tasteless, replacing it with other foods actually increases the flavor and variety of your diet. As you've seen, you can eat better than ever, and if you have to have starch, you can use the sugar-blocking foods you've learned about in this book to blunt its effects.

Now that you've learned how to recognize the culprits that cause sugar shocks and how to take advantage of the sugar-blocking effects of different foods, it's time to learn about other sugar-blocking techniques that will help you stabilize your blood sugar, reduce insulin demands, lose weight, and prevent or treat diabetes.

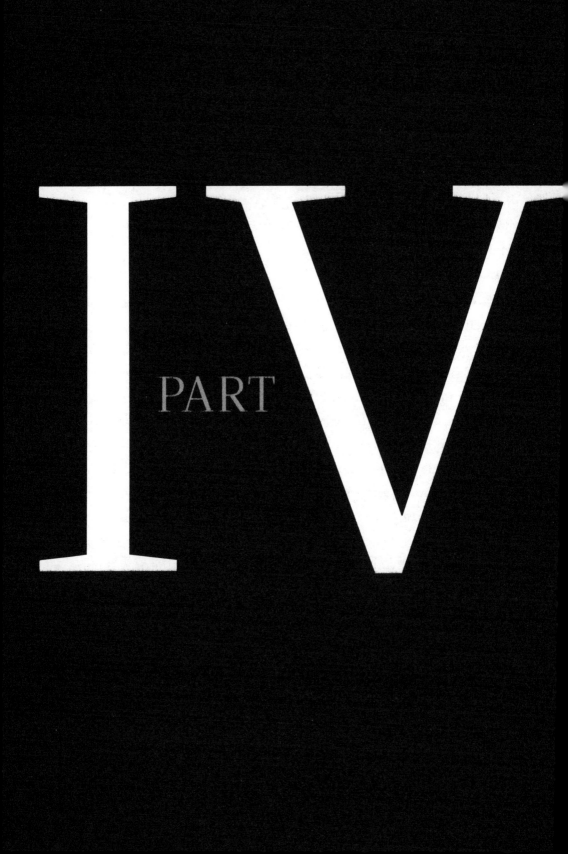

PART IV

SUGAR BLOCKERS: BEYOND DIET

THERE'S MORE TO THE EFFECTS of carbohydrates on your body than how many grams you eat. Much depends on what happens once glucose enters your bloodstream.

The stage for America's epidemic of obesity and diabetes was set by changes in patterns of physical activity that resulted in an epidemic of insulin resistance. In Chapter 11, you will learn how, by activating a particular type of muscle fiber called a slow-twitch fiber, you can, with minimal effort, target exercise specifically toward restoring insulin sensitivity and losing weight. Chapter 12 will help you coordinate sleep, work, and the kinds of meals you eat to improve the way your body handles carbohydrates. In Chapter 13, you will learn about newer sugar-blocking medications that not only prevent and treat diabetes but also produce significant and lasting weight loss in people with and without diabetes. Chapter 14 discusses what you need to do to prevent blood vessel disease, the number one killer and crippler of Americans.

11

EXERCISE:
GETTING THE MOST
BENEFIT WITH THE
LEAST EFFORT

THERE'S NO NEED TO PREACH—you know that exercise is good for you, not just for your body but also for your mind. Exercise is a natural antidepressant; it stimulates the same hormones as Prozac does. It relieves stress, calms your nerves, and improves your concentration and sleep. It arouses endorphins, your body's natural painkillers. If exercise were a drug, you couldn't keep people away from it.

Considering that exercise makes us feel so good and is so good for us, why don't we do it? It was fun when we were kids, but it seems that as we age, we develop an aversion to it. Exercise sounds good in the abstract—we remember how good it made us feel—but when it comes to actually doing it, all of a sudden we're struck by pangs of lethargy.

If grueling sessions of huffing and puffing don't appeal to you, you'll like what I'm about to tell you: Believe it or not, you have muscles in your body that don't cause fatigue when you exercise them. If you have a hard time believing that, think about your diaphragm, the muscle under the rib cage that powers your breathing. How tired does it get? It works continuously day and night, and you're not even aware of it. The reason your diaphragm never fatigues is that it's powered by a special kind of muscle fiber that does not run out of energy when you exercise it. Let me explain.

● SLOW-TWITCH FIBERS

You have two distinct kinds of muscle fibers in your body: type I, or slow-twitch, fibers, and type II, or fast-twitch, fibers. Both contain tiny power plants called mitochondria that use oxygen to replenish the energy they need to do their work. The difference is that slow-twitch fibers have many times more mitochondria than fast-twitch fibers do. Having lots of mitochondria allows them to use oxygen to replenish virtually all the energy they use *as they are working*. Because they don't build up an oxygen "debt," they don't have to rest.

In contrast, fast-twitch fibers contain few mitochondria. They are built to function for short bursts of intense activity without oxygen. However, they accumulate an oxygen debt, which must be repaid with periods of rest. That oxygen deficit causes the sense of fatigue you experience when you exercise a muscle.

Of course, your diaphragm is only a small portion of your total muscle mass. However, you have a much larger group of muscles powered by slow-twitch fibers: *your walking muscles*. They make up approximately 70 percent of your muscle mass, and like your diaphragm, they don't cause fatigue when you use them. Think about it: When you're walking at a normal pace—not pushing yourself, just trying to get from one place to another—do your leg muscles get tired? Be honest. Your feet might get sore, and you might get bored, or hot or cold, but are your muscles really tired? Most people can walk for hours without stopping. What other exercise could you do for that long without resting?

Every creature on Earth needs to breathe and get from point A to point B. Mother Nature was kind enough to make sure those essential activities were easy for us by powering our breathing and walking muscles with slow-twitch fibers. Exercise physiologists have found that of all the different types of activities we do, walking expends the most energy with the least *perceived* effort. It's hard to believe, but when you're walking, your muscles are working almost as hard as they would be if you were running; you just don't feel it.

Here's the secret to relieving insulin resistance: It turns out that those little energy-producing dynamos in your muscle cells—the mitochondria—are exactly what goes wrong when you have insulin resistance. What luck! Most of the mitochondria in your body are in your slow-twitch muscle fibers. That means that the muscles you need to exercise to relieve insulin resistance happen to be *the very ones that are the easiest to exercise.* You don't need to sweat and strain to relieve insulin resistance; all you need to do is walk.

How Fast, How Far, and How Often?

The metabolic pathways in your muscles that control their sensitivity to insulin behave as if they are controlled by a switch—they're turned either on or off. Walking turns the switch on, but you can't do it just by sauntering over to the watercooler. You have to do a little more exercise than that. However, once the switch is turned on, it's on. It doesn't do a lot of good to exercise more. Scientists have found that you can restore your muscles' sensitivity to insulin with as little as 20 minutes of walking. You get some added benefit by walking more, but not as much as you get in the first 20 minutes. Actually, distance is more important than time. Two miles will guarantee results. It doesn't matter whether you walk them or run them; the important thing is that you go the distance.

When it comes to preventing diabetes, research consistently shows that the difference between getting no exercise at all and walking just 20 minutes every other day is greater than the difference between walking regularly and being a long-distance runner. Think about what that means: It's not just that walking is good for you—you already knew that. It means that getting no exercise is *terrible for you.* If you don't exercise at all, you are decidedly less healthy than someone who walks just 20 minutes every other day.

Our bodies weren't made for sitting around. They were made for walking—that's their normal state—but a lot of us don't walk more than a couple of hundred feet a day. The fact is, if you're not walking regularly or doing some kind of exercise, you're a sick puppy. Lack of regular exercise raises your risk of diabetes, heart disease, and even some kinds of cancer.

How often do you need to exercise? When it comes to reducing insulin resistance, frequency, not intensity, is the key. Exercise restores your muscles' responsiveness to insulin for about 48 hours. After that, the switch turns off and your body shuts down to insulin. It doesn't matter if you run a marathon or walk a few miles; after 2 days you lose sensitivity to insulin. Just exercising on the weekends is not enough.

How fast do you need to move to turn on that switch? You need to walk as if you had to be somewhere at a certain time—as if you had an appointment to keep. If you were walking to work, for example, you wouldn't dillydally. You would give yourself enough time not to have to rush, but you would cover the distance as quickly as you comfortably could.

To see for yourself how muscles can work without fatigue, try this: After you've been walking for a while, pick up the pace to a level that makes you slightly uncomfortable—so that you can feel fatigue in your legs. Notice how aware you become of the work you're doing. The reason your legs feel tired is that your muscles are building up an oxygen debt. Now slow down a little. Do you see how quickly that fatigue subsides? That's the point at which the mitochondria in your slow-twitch muscles are completely replenishing the energy those muscles are using. At that speed you're getting the greatest amount of slow-twitch-muscle exercise with the least amount of effort. Your legs don't feel tired, and your mind moves on to other things.

Timing of Exercise

The time of day you choose to exercise doesn't matter much; what's important is that you do, indeed, exercise. No matter when you do it, moderate exercise such as walking immediately sensitizes your muscles to insulin

Remembering the Old Days

WHEN YOU were younger and slimmer, walking probably didn't seem like real exercise. Running—*that* was exercise! Maybe you're still in that mind-set. Wake up! Those days are gone. You're older and heavier now. Running isn't as easy as it was. That "bounce" in your running step is now a "thud." The reality is this: Not many people get back into running regularly after they've stopped for several years, entered middle age, and gained weight.

Question: What's the best thing about being overweight?

Answer: You have fantastic leg muscles. Carrying that extra weight around has given you big, strong calf, thigh, and buttock muscles. Get those puppies moving and they'll have a major impact on your metabolism. Since you have such big leg muscles, walking will probably increase your body's sensitivity to insulin more now than running did before, when those muscles were smaller.

and reduces after-meal blood sugar spikes for 24 to 48 hours afterward. Intense exercise—the kind that makes your heart race and leaves you gasping for breath—similarly improves insulin responsiveness. However, it can trigger an outpouring of adrenaline, which reduces your body's sensitivity to insulin for a couple of hours afterward. Very vigorous exercise immediately before a starchy meal can actually increase after-meal blood sugar levels.

As you exercise, channels open up in your muscle fibers that allow glucose to move from your bloodstream into your muscle cells *independent of insulin.* This unique effect starts as soon as you begin exercising and ends a few minutes after you stop. As mentioned in Chapter 7, a 20-minute walk immediately after a meal can reduce the after-meal blood sugar spike by half. If you can work it into your schedule, an after-meal hike is an effective sugar blocker.

● HUFFING AND PUFFING: WHAT'S THE POINT?

If you have the time and the energy to do more than walk for exercise, what kind of exercise should you do? This is worth thinking about because different types of exercise accomplish different things. Often people don't get as much benefit as they could from exercise because they aren't doing the right kind.

If your goal is to build endurance or stamina, you need to push yourself to the point of fatigue and maintain that level of exertion for several minutes or more. The longer and faster you go, the more endurance you build. On the other hand, if your goal is to build big muscles, you need a different approach. You need to strain your muscles against heavy resistance, as you do when you lift weights.

For the past 40 years, Americans have been fixated on endurance training, nicknamed cardio, as in *cardiovascular* endurance training. Running, cycling, and using a stair-climber or an elliptical trainer are all forms of this training. These days, when people think of exercising to lose weight, they usually think of endurance training.

When you engage in strenuous exercise such as running or using a stair-climber, you use largely the same muscles as when you walk, so you can similarly increase insulin sensitivity. However, anything that requires you to tolerate discomfort for long periods is, by definition, hard. Indeed, endurance training, which necessitates pushing yourself until you're huffing and puffing, demands willpower, energy, and motivation. The reality is that only a small minority of middle-aged folks do it regularly.

But you don't have to push yourself to the point of being uncomfortable to restore insulin sensitivity. You have to ask yourself, then, what are the advantages of endurance training over just walking for exercise? Running restores insulin sensitivity, but so does walking. Running increases the antidepressant hormone, but walking does, too. Endurance training helps you run faster and farther, but unless you're competing in races, why do you need to be able to run faster and farther? If you want to build strength, resistance exercise works better than endurance training. So what's the point of all the huffing and puffing?

The medical profession is at least partly to blame for America's fixation on endurance training. Before the 1960s, doctors thought that heart patients should avoid exertion. It was a revelation when researchers discovered that it was not only safe for most heart patients to exercise but also beneficial. A heart attack damages the pumping muscle of the heart and often results in limited endurance. Heart patients can often build their stamina back up with endurance training.

When word got out that endurance training was helping heart patients, others assumed that if it was good for heart patients, it must be good for everyone. Most people who are engaged in endurance training aren't recovering from a heart attack; they're hoping to *prevent* a heart attack.

Your endurance—for example, how far and how fast you can run—depends mainly on how fast your heart can pump blood. Endurance training enables your heart to pump more blood with each beat. However, heart attacks are not caused by a weak heart muscle. They're caused by blockages of the arteries that lead to the heart muscle. Having a strong heart muscle will not keep you from getting blocked arteries.

Research shows that if your goal is to lose weight, lower blood sugar, and prevent heart disease, walking for exercise is almost as good as running, and it's certainly a lot easier to do—especially for those middle-aged and older. Indeed, initiating a running program after not exercising for several years is a notorious way to cause musculoskeletal injuries. The only physical benefit that endurance training provides over walking is that you can run longer distances in shorter amounts of time—useful for winning foot races but otherwise low on most people's list of priorities. Remember, walking also strengthens your heart muscle and builds endurance. When you're walking, you're expending almost as much energy as when you're running. You just don't feel it because you're using those type 1, or slow-twitch, muscle fibers.

Some people throw themselves into running because they think that using their leg and buttock muscles will selectively remove fat from those areas. It doesn't work that way. Exercising a particular part of your body will not remove any more fat from that part than exercising some other part of your body. In fact, exercise of any kind tends to remove more fat from your abdomen than from other places.

A few years ago, I saw a photograph of a dozen or so Seattle business-men taken in 1915. They were all wearing shirts and ties, so they weren't doing physical labor all day. It struck me that there wasn't an overweight one in the bunch. I asked myself, What did they do differently that kept them slim? At the turn of the 20th century, people actually ate more than we do now. They didn't belong to health clubs. The only physical activity I could think of that they did more of then than we do now is walk. In those days, Seattle's business district was a mile or two from most of the residential parts of town, and people thought nothing of walking a few miles to get to work. They also walked at their jobs more than we do. They didn't have e-mail. If they needed to talk to somebody, they did it face-to-face.

Shortly thereafter, I gave up my expensive downtown parking place and started walking to work. I have been doing it for 5 years now. I'm surprised by how much I enjoy it. I lost 20 pounds and have never gained it back.

As test panelist Jane Wilchak urged: "Just go for a walk; it's as easy as that. Don't exercise if you don't want to, but everyone can go for a walk."

● THE NEXT STEP

If you already walk or jog regularly and you have the energy and time to do more, rather than trying to build more endurance, from the standpoint of your health you would benefit more by building muscle strength. Although walking and running are effective for losing weight and preventing diabetes, they don't build much muscle mass. For that, you need resistance exercise.

Resistance exercise requires you to exert force against resistance—the kind of exercise you do when you lift weights. It's the best way to build muscle mass. Remember that your muscles are your main consumers of glucose, and the target of most of the insulin your body produces. The more muscle you have, the better your insulin will work. Whereas walking or running restores insulin sensitivity for a couple of days, increasing your muscle mass has a permanent effect. Muscle removes glucose from your bloodstream even while you sleep, and the more muscle you have, the more glucose it removes. And recent research has found that resistance exercise adds to the insulin-sensitizing effects of walking.

When you were younger—under age 30—it didn't take much exercise to build up your muscles. Indeed, a 30-year-old can look buff even without regular exercise. But once you turn 40, it's as if someone flipped a switch. Your muscle mass spontaneously starts dwindling away. If you don't exercise, you lose about 8 percent of your muscle mass every decade after age 40. The good news is that resistance exercise can prevent age-related loss of muscle mass.

Some people, especially women, shy away from muscle-strengthening exercise because they think it will make them appear muscle-bound. Don't worry; after age 30, you can't build muscle as easily as you could when you were younger. This is particularly true of women, because they don't have as much of the muscle-building hormone testosterone in their systems as men do. Instead, muscle-strengthening exercise gives your muscles "definition"—it restores their natural shape and keeps them from looking flabby.

You may think that because you're already toughening up your legs by walking or running, you won't benefit much by trying to strengthen them further with resistance exercise. To some extent, that's true; walking and running will strengthen your legs. However, recall the other kind of muscle fiber: the type 2, or fast-twitch, fibers. When you walk or run, you exercise mainly your slow-twitch fibers. Your fast-twitch fibers don't get much of a workout. Resistance exercise activates those type 2 fibers, which gives your legs more power, makes walking easier, and improves your balance. Your leg and buttock muscles are the largest muscles in your body. Because of their mere size, they contribute more to insulin sensitivity than other muscle groups do. Although type 2 muscle fibers aren't as important as type 1 fibers for restoring insulin sensitivity, exercising them does add to the effects of walking or running.

Crafting a Strength-Training Regimen

The effectiveness of resistance exercise in building muscle strength depends not on the number of times a muscle contracts but on the force against which it contracts. Exercise physiologists have found that you can actually strengthen a muscle by doing just one contraction a week, as long as it's against maximal resistance. Conversely, repetitively contracting a muscle against light resistance has little strengthening effect. Experts recommend doing two sets of 10 to 12 repetitions each, with the final exertion of the second set done against maximal resistance. You can determine maximal resistance by increasing resistance until you can't do 10 repetitions, then reducing the resistance to the point at which you barely can. For example, if you can lift 25 pounds 10 times, but you can't do the same with 27.5 pounds—the next-heaviest weight available—25 pounds would be your maximum.

For muscle strengthening, there's no need to exercise continuously. You can catch your breath and rest between sets. You can even break up your workout, if you prefer, and do one set in the morning and one set in the evening. Two or three exercise sessions a week is enough to get results. Give yourself a day between sessions to allow your muscles time to recover.

The more muscles you exercise, the greater the beneficial effects on your body's sensitivity to insulin. A good insulin-sensitizing program includes exercises that strengthen all of the major muscle groups of your body. Think about it this way: You have two sets of muscles for each joint— muscles that bend, or "flex," the joint, and ones that straighten, or "extend," it. To get the most benefit, you need to exercise the muscles that flex and extend all of your major joints—elbows, shoulders, hips, and knees—as well as your torso.

Joining a full-service gym is a good investment in your health. However, you can put together a good muscle-strengthening routine with some dumbbells, a resistance band, and a bench.

If you haven't done strength training before, here are some basics. The term *rep* is short for repetition: For instance, each time you lift and lower a dumbbell, it's a repetition. A series of reps is called a set.

Try to choose weights that will allow you to complete 10 reps but make you feel as if you couldn't do an 11th. If you can't do at least 8 reps, go for a lighter weight; if you feel that you could do 12 or more, pick a heavier one.

Resistance bands or tubes add more flexibility to your routine. Unlike dumbbells, they keep the tension on the entire time and in all kinds of directions; they are also light and easy to bring with you when you travel. You can choose either a flat band or a tube with handles. Bands and

WHEN YOU DON'T FEEL Like Exercising

IF YOU sometimes find yourself lacking in motivation, I suggest that you have two kinds of workout routines: one for when you're full of energy, and one for when you're not. If you have the energy, do a full workout—go to a gym or take an ambitious walk or run. However, for those times when your ambition seems to leave you, have an easier, fallback routine, maybe just a 20-minute walk. Remember, when it comes to reducing insulin resistance and treating or preventing diabetes, the frequency of exercise—not intensity—is key. And the difference between walking 20 minutes a day and being a couch potato is huge.

Once you get into a routine and experience the benefits of exercise, you may find that you want to exercise more. As tester Michelle Newhard put it: "I never thought I could fit it in before, but now I can work out 1½ hours every day if I want to! I love working out!"

tubes come in a variety of resistances. As you progress, you can increase resistance simply by shortening the band.

Some of the exercises in this chapter call for a weight bench. If you don't have one, you can use an ottoman or a stability ball—an inflated exercise ball. Stability balls add an extra balance challenge to exercise. Choose a size that allows you to sit with your feet flat and your thighs about parallel to the floor. The more inflated and the firmer the ball, the harder it is to balance on it.

Lower-back pain is the number one orthopedic complaint of middle-aged and older folks. Situps are one of the best exercises for preventing lower-back injuries. To prepare your lower back for exercise, do situps before you start your other exercises.

SITUPS

1. Lie on your back with your knees bent, feet flat on the floor, and hands behind your head.

2. Exhale as you sit up and curl your torso toward your thighs. Continue curling up until your head is as close to your knees as possible.

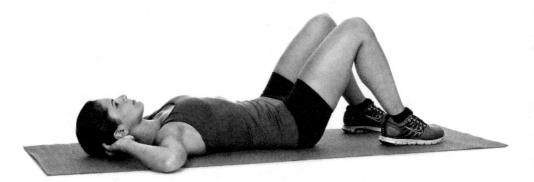

3. Inhale and slowly lower your torso back toward the floor in a controlled fashion, keeping your feet, tailbone, and lower back in contact with the mat.

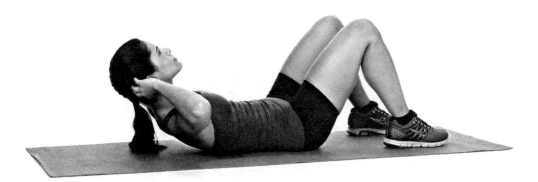

BICEPS CURL

1. Sit on a bench, a sturdy chair, or a stability ball, with your feet planted firmly on the floor. You should have a dumbbell in each hand, with your palms facing forward. (You can also do this exercise standing if you prefer.)

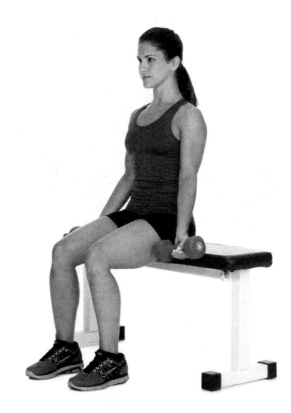

2. Exhale and slowly bend one elbow at a time, bringing the dumbbells toward your chest without arching your back or moving your elbows forward.

3. Inhale and gently lower the dumbbells to the starting position.

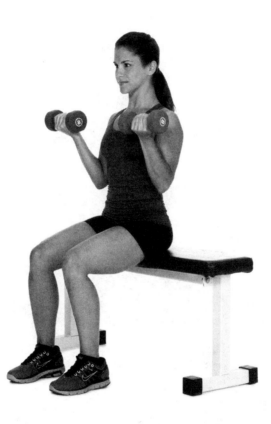

CHEST PRESS

1. Sit on a bench, a sturdy chair, or a stability ball, with your feet planted firmly on the floor. Hold a dumbbell in each hand on either side of your shoulders, palms facing forward.

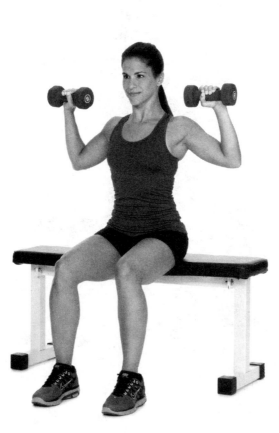

2. Exhale and press the dumbbells overhead in unison until your elbows are fully extended. Don't arch your back, and keep your shoulders down.

3. Inhale and slowly lower the weights back to the starting position.

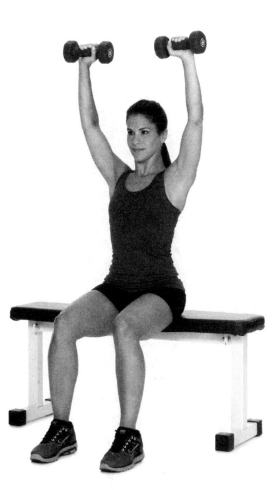

SHOULDER SHRUG

1. Stand with your feet hip-width apart, your arms at your sides, a dumbbell in each hand, and your palms facing your body.

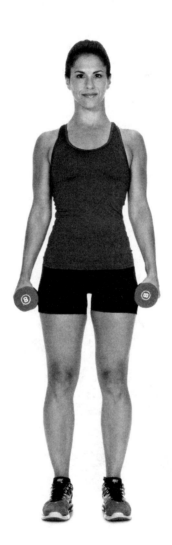

2. Exhale and slowly shrug your shoulders upward. Avoid rotating your shoulders, arching your back, and bending your elbows or wrists.

3. Inhale and slowly lower the dumbbells back to the starting position.

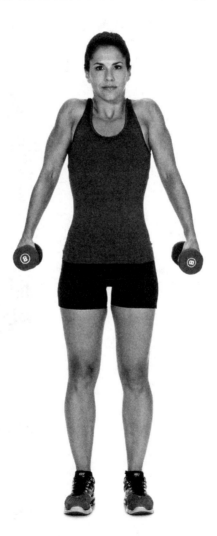

TRICEPS PULLDOWN

1. Wrap a resistance band around an anchor point above your head. Stand with one foot slightly in front of the other, with either end of the band in each hand, your palms facing the floor. Your elbows should be bent, with your forearms nearly parallel to the floor.

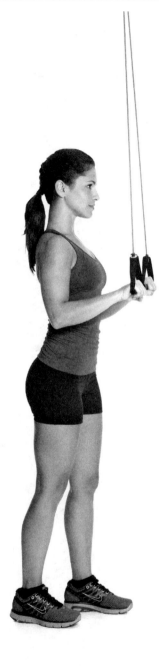

2. Exhale and slowly extend or straighten your elbows. Avoid moving your upper arms, and don't bend your wrists.

3. Inhale and slowly return your arms to the starting position.

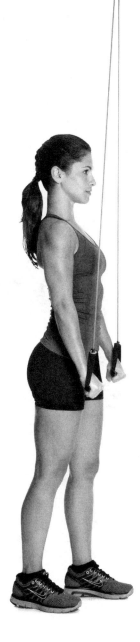

CHEST FLY

1. Holding a dumbbell in each hand, with your palms facing each other, lie on your back on a flat bench, an ottoman, or a stability ball, with your feet planted firmly on the floor. If you are using a chair or a ball, make sure that your head and upper back are supported. Your arms should be level with your shoulders or your chest, with elbows extended and not locked.

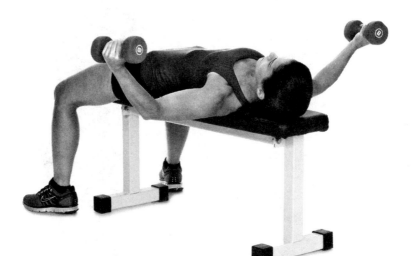

2. Exhale and slowly raise the dumbbells upward in a wide arc until they almost meet at the top. Keep your elbows bent, as if you were hugging a big beach ball.

3. Inhale and slowly lower the dumbbells back to the starting position.

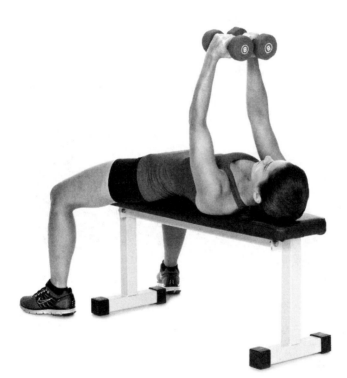

SEATED ROW

1. Wrap a resistance band or tube securely around a sturdy piece of furniture, like a sofa leg. Sit on the floor with your knees slightly bent and hold either end of the band in each hand.

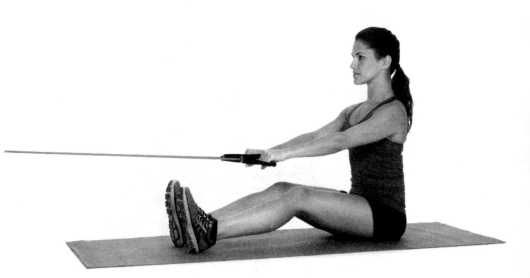

2. Without leaning backward, exhale and pull the band toward you, bending your elbows. Avoid arching your back and shrugging your shoulders.

3. Inhale and gently extend your elbows back to the starting position.

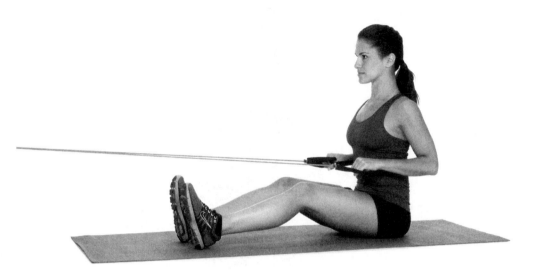

LEG LIFT

1. Stand with your feet together and your hands on your hips.

2. Exhale and slowly lift one leg about 3 to 6 inches off the floor. Hold for 15 seconds.

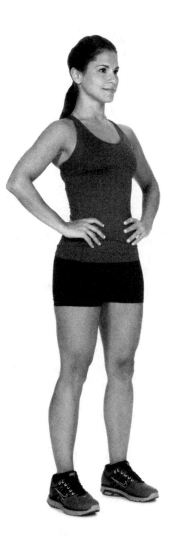

3. Inhale and return your raised foot to the floor. Switch sides and perform an equal number of reps on each leg.

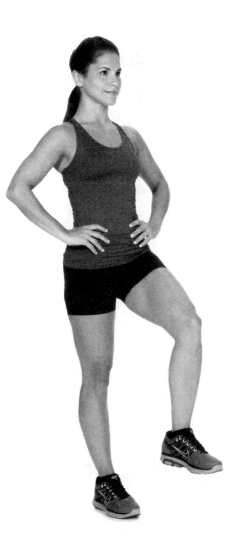

SQUAT

1. Stand with your feet slightly wider than hip width apart, your hands at your sides.

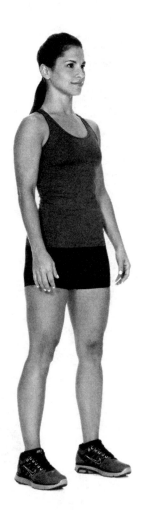

2. Stiffen your core and abdominal muscles, hold your chest up, shift your weight back into your heels, and slowly bend your knees and lower your hips as if you were about to sit in a chair. Make sure that your knees stay over your toes.

3. Exhale and return to the starting position.

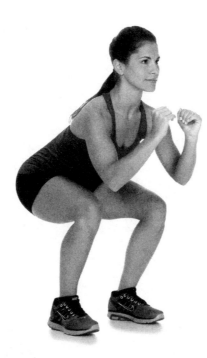

HAMSTRING CURL

1. Wrap a resistance band or tube securely around a sturdy piece of furniture, like a sofa leg. Tie the other end to one ankle. Stand with your feet about hip-width apart.

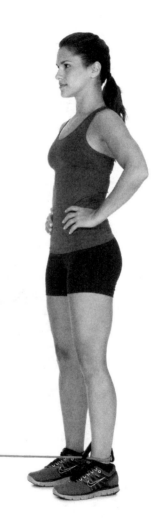

2. Slowly lift the foot with the band off the floor. Exhale, then curl or bend your knee, bringing your heel toward your buttock without moving your thigh.

3. Inhale and slowly lower your leg to the starting position.

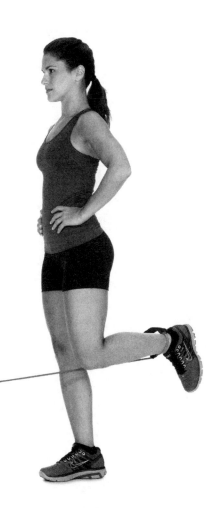

12

BLOCKING THE SUGAR THAT COMES FROM WITHIN

YOUR BODY is very adept at changing the food you eat to whatever nutrient it needs. It has no trouble converting glucose to fat or fat back to glucose. If you haven't eaten for a few hours, your liver converts fat and protein to glucose to keep your blood sugar up. However, if you have insulin resistance or diabetes, your liver can work against you. If its timing is off—if it produces glucose when glucose is not needed, such as immediately after meals—glucose coming from your liver adds to the glucose in the food you eat and worsens after-meal blood sugar spikes.

● THE STRESS-SUGAR LINK

Although your body's sensitivity to insulin is mainly a matter of how physically active you are, it can be influenced by other things, particularly the hormone adrenaline. Adrenaline is the fight-or-flight hormone; it prepares you for physical exertion. As it courses through your system, it makes your heart pump harder, tenses your muscles, and puts you in an anxious state of mind, vaguely aware of the possibility of danger. Mother Nature gave us this reflex to protect us from physical threats of the type that prehistoric humans encountered—saber-toothed tigers and such. However, these days the usual causes of adrenaline surges are not physical threats; they're those nerve-jangling mental experiences such as work frustrations, confrontations with other humans, and time pressure.

In addition to its other actions, adrenaline opposes the action of insulin on the liver. Whereas insulin transports glucose out of your blood and into your liver, adrenaline moves glucose in the opposite direction: out of your liver and into your blood. That's fine if the adrenaline surge is followed by vigorous physical action, as nature intended. Your muscles use the extra glucose for energy. But if you're just sitting at your desk getting your nerves jangled, all this does is raise your blood sugar. If you eat starch or sugar during an adrenaline surge, your blood sugar will rise higher than it would otherwise.

Of course, stress is a fact of life. If there were anything you could do about it, you would already be doing it. However, you don't have to eliminate stress to reduce the effects of adrenaline on your blood sugar. You can benefit by just avoiding it during meals. Thankfully, adrenaline doesn't stay long in your bloodstream. A few minutes of relaxation will allow it to settle down while you eat. Taking time to relax at mealtimes—getting away from the hustle and bustle of the office or enjoying some light conversation—is not only pleasant but also better for your health. Sure, you could wolf down lunch at your desk between phone calls. But maybe there's a reason we have a lunch *hour*.

● SLEEP AND INSULIN SENSITIVITY

Sleep has profound effects on insulin sensitivity. Researchers have discovered that just 2 nights of bad sleep measurably worsen insulin resistance. A survey of 87,000 people conducted by the National Center for Health Statistics found that 33 percent of responders who said they slept less than 6 hours a night were obese. Those who reported sleeping 7 to 8 hours per night were slimmer—only 22 percent were obese. Bad sleep has also been linked to a higher risk of type 2 diabetes. In a study, University of Chicago researchers suppressed deep sleep in a group of healthy young adults. After just 3 nights of deep-sleep suppression, the subjects became less sensitive to insulin by an amount comparable to that caused by gaining 20 to 30 pounds.

As with stress, if there were anything you could do to get a better night's sleep, you would probably be doing it. Nevertheless, at times when you can't get adequate sleep, such as when you're working long hours or traveling, you should take special care to maintain your sensitivity to insulin by exercising, avoiding high–glycemic load foods, and using your sugar-blocking skills.

Your Body Clock and Your Blood Sugar

When it comes to your health, the regularity of your sleep is as important as—and possibly more important than—the total amount you get. Many of the body's systems fluctuate rhythmically in 24-hour-long cycles including adrenaline levels, hormones, body temperature, the blood's tendency to clot, and, particularly, your body's sensitivity to insulin.

Like the conductor of an orchestra, a center in your brain—the supra-chiasmatic nucleus, or SCN—synchronizes all of those systems. Scientists call the coordinated cycling of various physiological systems the circadian rhythm, or body clock.

Your body clock synchronizes itself to darkness and light. When you wake in the morning, light hitting your eyes activates your SCN, and your internal timer starts ticking. It makes you alert and energetic during waking hours and sleepy when it's time to rest.

Of course, prehistoric humans had no lanterns or lightbulbs. Their body clocks were synchronized according to the rising and setting of the sun—they moved about during the day and slept at night. Now, thanks to artificial light, we don't have to abide by the cycles of the sun as most other creatures do. We can stay up at night and sleep during the day.

Whenever you change your sleep schedule—say, if you're accustomed to working days, and then you start working nights—it takes several days for your body clock to adjust. Meanwhile, you're awake when your body clock thinks you should be sleeping, and when you have to sleep, it thinks you should be awake.

Scientists have discovered that being out of sync with your body clock reduces your body's sensitivity to insulin. For example, among night-shift workers, meals consumed in the middle of the night raise blood sugar more than those eaten at the usual times. Indeed, insulin resistance, obesity, and diabetes are more common in night-shift workers than in those working only day shifts.

Air travel causes a similar problem: jet lag. Like workers on the night shift, travelers who cross time zones often find themselves awake when their bodies think they should be asleep, and vice versa. The main manifestations of jet lag are fits of sleepiness during the day and insomnia at night. And evidence suggests that jet lag, like shift work, lowers insulin resistance.

Probably the most common circadian-rhythm disturbance is a pattern of sleeping and waking that regular daytime workers often get into. During the workweek, 9-to-5'ers frequently get behind in their sleep and then sleep late on the weekend. Delaying your wake-up time by sleeping in an hour or two on weekends is enough to reset your body clock forward. Then, when it's time to go back to work on Monday, you have trouble falling asleep at night and waking up in the morning. Sleep specialists call this the delayed sleep-phase syndrome, and like jet lag, it's linked to reduced insulin sensitivity and increased after-meal blood sugar levels.

Sleep Apnea

Apnea is a medical term for temporary stoppage of breathing. A lot of people periodically stop breathing during sleep, which is called sleep apnea. Actually, most of us have occasional apnea while we sleep; it's not uncommon to stop breathing for a few seconds. However, some individuals do it excessively. Apnea spells can last 15 to 20 seconds and occur as often as 40 to 50 times an hour.

The Caffeine Conundrum

HERE'S A PUZZLER FOR YOU: Caffeine is known to boost adrenalin levels, which raise blood sugar. However, more than one research study has found that heavy coffee drinkers are less likely to develop diabetes. What to make of this apparent contradiction?

A review of the research doesn't help much. A few studies have found that a moderate amount of coffee may lower the risk for diabetes. However, some smaller studies have linked caffeine to higher blood sugar levels after meals. The only reasonable conclusion you can make is that, when it comes to caffeine's effect on blood sugar, the jury's still out.

Then, in 2010, researchers conducted a meta-analysis of studies that examined the association between caffeine consumption and the risk of diabetes. This included a 2005 study that incorporated findings on nearly 200,000 participants. This study suggested that consuming six or seven cups of coffee per day reduces a person's risk of diabetes by about a third. A couple cups of coffee a day probably won't hurt you and is a better choice than soda or juice.

Sleep apnea rarely poses any immediate danger. However, it can prevent you from getting the right kind of sleep. You may think you sleep well, but you're not getting enough of what's called restorative sleep—the deep sleep that replenishes your energy and alertness. Consequently, you suffer from excessive sleepiness and tiredness during the day.

Obesity brings on sleep apnea, which is why America is now experiencing an epidemic of sleep apnea. Of course, obesity is linked to insulin resistance, so people with sleep apnea often have insulin resistance. On the other hand, sleep apnea causes your body to produce more adrenaline at night, which further reduces insulin sensitivity. Thus, obesity sets the stage for sleep apnea, which lowers insulin sensitivity, which promotes more weight gain.

Sometimes doctors recommend treatment of sleep apnea with small home respirators called continuous positive airway pressure, or CPAP, devices. These machines deliver a steady stream of compressed air to your airways via a hose attached to a face mask. The flow of air keeps your airway open so that you can get the restorative sleep you need. Besides improving insulin resistance, CPAP treatment can dramatically improve daytime sleepiness and energy levels. Exercise and weight loss also improve sleep apnea—and the insulin resistance that goes along with it.

● TURNING OFF THE SUGAR TAP

If you have sleep problems—due to shift changes, jet lag, insomnia, or sleep apnea—correcting them will improve your body's sensitivity to insulin and help reduce those after-meal sugar shocks. However, if you can't find a solution to your sleep problem, it's even more important to reduce the glycemic load of your diet and to use sugar blockers to inhibit the absorption of glucose into your bloodstream.

The best way to counteract the effects of stress, irregular hours, and a lack of restorative sleep on insulin sensitivity is by exercising. Your muscles are your main users of glucose and the target of most of the insulin you produce. Exercising overrides those negative effects and resensitizes your body to insulin.

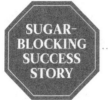
CINDY SWAN
From Can't Keep Up to Hard to Catch

Age: 59

Height: 5' 5"

Pounds lost: 10

Inches lost: 11

Major accomplishment: Lost 11" and almost as many pounds!

Favorite sugar blockers: Wine before dinner and chia seeds on salads

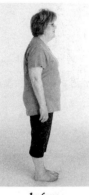

before

CINDY SWAN AND HER FAMILY used to like to eat out on weekends. Then she started eating the Sugar Blockers Diet way . . . and they still do! "I didn't have to change that," said Cindy, who lost 11 inches (and almost as many pounds) on the program. "You just think about what you're ordering, have a glass of wine. . . . It was just easy," she said of continuing her weekend nights out on the town. And Cindy added that no one dining with her would have known that she was on a "diet," because it didn't feel like one!

In the past, she had tried plenty of other weight loss programs. In those, Cindy said, you had to watch points, pay for the program, buy its supplements and bars, and eat so many of the bars a day. The Sugar Blockers Diet "is all regular food you can buy in a grocery store and that you'd buy anyway. You're buying fresh fruits and vegetables." It was easy—a few little tricks that anyone can do, she explained. "It's amazing that it's so simple. I even had pizza; just didn't eat the crust. I didn't feel like I was sacrificing anything."

Beforehand, Cindy's biggest problem came after work. As an occupational health nurse, she has an early start to her workday, which automatically makes eating normal meals difficult. "When I got home at 3:00, I'd be hungry after [having had] lunch at 11:00," she said. "That's when my worst time was. I'd snack on bad things," which didn't help her weight or her health. (Cindy had been diagnosed as prediabetic.) These days, though, she is not so hungry when she gets home, and if she is (that's allowed!), she knows exactly what to reach for. "I'll have almonds and a piece of fruit—almonds fill you up," Cindy said, adding that throughout the day she feels satisfied. She's satisfied with her health measures, too. Her postmeal blood sugar spikes are declining more and more each week, and a consistent diet and regular exercise are leading to a leaner, healthier Cindy.

On top of knowing the right things to eat, Cindy discovered that just a bit of walking can work wonders. "I have had sciatic pain, and I don't notice it as much with the walking," she said. She increased the amount of walking and weight training as each week went on and found many of the suggested Sugar Blockers Diet exercises both easy to fit into her schedule and easy to do. "You have more flexibility just from moving more."

Shortly after starting the program, Cindy bought a 5-pound weight. "When you pick up a 5-pound weight and think [about how] your body is carrying around 10 extra of those [pounds] . . . after I lost the first 5 pounds, I realized, Whoa, I don't have to carry those extra 5 pounds anymore," she said. Watching the weight come off motivated her to keep going. Just a few weeks after the official end of the program, she had lost 4 more pounds.

When Cindy first decided to give the Sugar Blockers Diet a try, an upcoming trip to the Grand Canyon was her motivating factor—she wanted to be in better shape so that she could go on hikes with her family and "not feel like the slug that's holding them back." Now that she's leaner, lighter, and a regular walker, they may have to worry about keeping up with her!

after

13

SUGAR-BLOCKING MEDICATIONS AND **WEIGHT LOSS**

I F YOU REDUCE the glycemic load of your diet and restore your muscles' sensitivity to insulin with exercise, you should steadily lose weight. But the fact is that efforts to change our diet and exercise habits sometimes don't work. Some folks are genetically more prone to insulin resistance than others; they don't have the time or energy, or ability, to exercise; or, whether by force of habit or by hormonal quirk, they have trouble eliminating refined carbohydrates. If you just can't seem to make any progress, there is another option: medication.

Take a drug to lose weight? Drugs are for diseases, right? Well, if obesity isn't a disease, what is? It brings on diabetes, heart disease, arthritis, infertility in women, even some kinds of cancer. It disables you, discourages you, spoils your looks, and shortens your life. That's not a disease?

If you're a veteran of the battle of the bulge, you've no doubt heard about a lot of diet pills over the years, from Fen-Phen (fenfluramine and phentermine) to Meridia (sibutramine) to Xenical and Alli (orlistat). You may even have tried a few. By now you're probably skeptical that any medication really works—and with good reason. It was always the same story: You would lose a few pounds, but within a few weeks you would gain them back, whether or not you continued taking the drug. Some of the drugs had serious side effects. None did anything to alleviate the underlying problem of insulin resistance and excessive insulin secretion.

I'm here to tell you that it's a new day. Doctors can now prescribe medications that safely produce significant weight loss that lasts. Considering that obesity and type 2 diabetes are just different manifestations of the same disease, it's not surprising that these medications were developed to treat type 2 diabetes. However, they are increasingly being used to treat obesity in people without diabetes.

What these medications have in common is that they all reduce the body's demands for insulin, and they are all *sugar blockers*. As diabetes medications, they lower blood sugar, but they also improve many of the other problems that come along with type 2 diabetes, including cholesterol imbalance, high blood pressure, overactive blood clotting, and blood vessel damage. Unlike older drugs that spurred the body to produce more insulin and made people gain weight, these medications reduce insulin demands and promote weight loss.

These new sugar-blocking medications were developed to combat insulin resistance in diabetics, but as you know, diabetics aren't the only ones whose bodies are resistant to insulin. Most chubby folks are just as insulin resistant. Many overweight individuals make five or six times the normal amounts of insulin to overcome their bodies' loss of sensitivity to it. Just as with type 2 diabetes, excessive insulin drives calories into fat stores, creates a state of internal starvation, and causes weight gain.

Once doctors realized that obesity and type 2 diabetes are just different manifestations of the same underlying physiological disturbances, they started asking the obvious question: If medications that reduce insulin demands lead to weight loss in type 2 diabetics, why wouldn't they help folks *without* diabetes lose weight? Why wait until excessive insulin demands cause your beta cells to wear out and your blood sugar levels to rise? Why not get started early, take advantage of the weight loss effects of these medications, and avoid diabetes? Indeed, researchers have recently tested these drugs on overweight people without diabetes and found that they not only promote weight loss, improve cholesterol balance, and lower blood pressure but actually prevent diabetes.

So far, the FDA has approved these medications only to treat type 2 diabetes. Nevertheless, as with many FDA-approved drugs, doctors are now prescribing these medications "off-label" to help their overweight and prediabetic patients lose weight and avoid diabetes.

None of these medications is a magic bullet. However, teaming the Sugar Blockers Program with medication can be a winning combination. When Debbie, a patient of mine for several years, reached her late forties, she started gaining weight despite her best efforts to diet and exercise. As many women that age do, she developed signs of insulin resistance: Her triglyceride level rose, her blood pressure went up, and her good-cholesterol level fell. Although she didn't have diabetes, I suggested that she try taking two of these new sugar-blocking medications. Within a few months she was back to her old weight, and the signs of insulin resistance disappeared.

Make no mistake: Debbie didn't just let the medications do the work. She also continued doing her best to exercise and to avoid high–glycemic load foods, but for her, medications made a big difference.

● ACARBOSE

As you learned in Chapter 4, acarbose is a natural substance produced by soil bacteria. It slows carbohydrate digestion by inhibiting amylase, the enzyme that breaks down starch to sugar in your small intestine. The huge amounts of amylase that your pancreas secretes when you eat carbohydrates are more suited to a diet of bark and roots than to the easily digestible carbohydrates that we modern humans eat. Acarbose puts amylase back in balance with the kinds of foods we eat.

Acarbose reduces the blood sugar spike that occurs after a carbohydrate-containing meal by as much as 30 to 40 percent. In the STOP-NIDDM study mentioned in Chapter 4, subjects who took acarbose lost weight following the same diet as the comparison-group members, who gained weight. By lowering the body's demands for insulin, acarbose not only improves blood sugar control in people who have diabetes but can actually prevent diabetes in people at risk of developing it. In addition, acarbose improves cholesterol balance and lowers blood pressure, and it has been proved to reduce the risk of heart attack.

Acarbose is by far the safest antidiabetes medication you can take. It actually works "outside" the body—it passes through your intestines without entering your bloodstream. Because acarbose lowers the body's demands for insulin, people with diabetes who take insulin shots need to be careful when starting it to avoid low blood sugar. For that reason you still need a doctor's prescription to obtain acarbose. The brand name is Precose, but it's also widely available as an inexpensive generic medication.

Acarbose works better for inhibiting the absorption of starch than of sugar. Sugar is digested by other enzymes besides amylase, which acarbose does not inhibit.

The only common side effect of acarbose is gassiness. Acarbose causes refined carbs to behave the way unrefined carbs in your intestinal tract do—like fresh fruits and vegetables. Acarbose inhibits starch digestion, so when undigested starch reaches the colon, where bacteria break it down, gas is released, similar to what happens when people abruptly increase their intake of fresh fruits and vegetables.

Your intestinal tract soon adapts to more slowly absorbed carbohydrates. The gassiness from acarbose, as well as from eating fruit and vegetables, subsides in a week or so. You're less likely to experience gassiness if you're used to eating lots of fresh fruit and vegetables. You can avoid the medication's side effects if you start with a small dose and increase it over the course of a few weeks.

● METFORMIN

If you have diabetes, metformin (pharmaceutical name: Glucophage) is the medication that most diabetes specialists suggest you take first. As you recall from Chapter 4, your liver is the first organ to receive blood coming from your small intestine. It's supposed to take up glucose after you eat and put it back into your bloodstream between meals. If you're insulin resistant, your liver secretes glucose into your bloodstream even as your intestine is absorbing it from food. This worsens after-meal blood sugar spikes and drives up insulin demands. Metformin helps the liver absorb glucose, which blunts blood sugar spikes and reduces your body's need for insulin. In addition to lowering blood sugar, metformin improves cholesterol balance, lowers blood pressure, and promotes weight loss.

Weight loss from metformin usually amounts to only a pound or two if there is no attempt to change lifestyle. A review of several studies that was published in the *International Journal of Obesity* in 2008 found that metformin resulted in weight loss in only about half of the studies examined. However, if you combine metformin with a low–glycemic load diet, the effects can be dramatic. In a study reported in the journal *Obesity,* Saint Louis University researchers put two groups of subjects with type 2 diabetes on the same weight loss diet. They treated one group with metformin and the other with a dummy pill that looked like metformin. After 6 months, those in the group that took metformin along with the diet lost an average of 17 more pounds than did the group that took the placebo.

Most of the medications that doctors used in the past for treating diabetes raised insulin levels but did not alleviate insulin resistance. While lowering blood sugar by increasing insulin levels helps prevent small–blood vessel damage—the cause of eye and kidney damage—it does not prevent large–blood vessel damage, the cause of heart attacks and strokes. Metformin was the first diabetes medication proved to prevent large-blood vessel damage. One of the largest, most carefully controlled studies on diabetes, the United Kingdom Prospective Diabetes Study, showed that metformin not only helps prevent small–blood vessel damage but also

WEIGHT LOSS HORMONES: Incretins

THE ACTIONS of the organ systems in your body that handle nutrients—including your stomach, intestines, pancreas, and liver—are tightly coordinated by nerve circuits and hormones. Several of these digestive hormones serve to regulate sugar absorption— they slow its absorption into your bloodstream. Among these is a group of hormones called incretins, which are secreted by clusters of cells in the walls of your small intestine in response to carbohydrates.

One of these hormones, gastric inhibitory peptide (GIP), acts on the pyloric valve at the outlet of the stomach to inhibit stomach emptying.

Another, glucagon-like peptide-1 (GLP-1), has several sugar-blocking effects.

Scientists have discovered that obese people, as well as people with type 2 diabetes, have diminished incretin activity, which causes them to digest food more rapidly than normal. This results in elevated after-meal blood sugar levels, rapid return of hunger between meals, and a tendency to gain weight.

Restoring incretin activity with medications that mimic these hormones slows digestion, blunts after-meal blood sugar spikes, reduces insulin needs, and promotes weight loss.

---

reduces the incidence of heart attacks. (As it turns out, acarbose also prevents heart attacks, but this wasn't known at the time.)

Metformin not only treats diabetes but can actually prevent it. By reducing the body's demands for insulin, metformin reduces the burden on the beta cells and keeps them from wearing out. In a study called the Diabetes Prevention Program, reported in the *New England Journal of Medicine,* researchers gave metformin to more than a thousand people who were at increased risk of developing diabetes. In 3 years, metformin had reduced the diabetes rate by 31 percent.

Doctors also use metformin to treat polycystic ovary syndrome (PCOS), another condition caused by insulin resistance. PCOS is the leading cause of infertility among women. It leads to obesity, irregular menstruation, abnormal hair growth, and an increased risk of diabetes. Metformin not only lowers the risk of diabetes in women with PCOS but also restores normal periods and fertility.

The only common side effect of metformin is diarrhea, which occurs when metformin doesn't get completely absorbed in the intestine. Some metformin reaches the colon, where it irritates the lining. Diarrhea subsides promptly when you stop taking the medication. You can avoid diarrhea by reducing the dose or taking metformin with food. Rarely, metformin causes acid buildup in the blood. This mainly occurs in people with sluggish kidney function caused by kidney disease. You should have a blood test to make sure that your kidneys work well before taking metformin.

● GLP-1 ANALOGS: POTENT WEIGHT LOSS HORMONES

Although acarbose and metformin promote weight loss, unless you're also watching your diet and exercising, the effects are modest. However, a new category of sugar-blocking medications has recently become popular that has much more powerful weight loss effects. These medications, called GLP-1 analogs, mimic a natural hormone produced by your small intestine called glucagon-like peptide-1 (GLP-1).

When carbohydrates reach your intestine, cells in the intestinal lining secrete GLP-1 into the bloodstream. GLP-1 keeps glucose from rushing into your system too fast and raising your blood sugar. It works as a sugar blocker on several parts of the digestive system at once. It slows stomach emptying, helps your liver take up glucose, and causes insulin to be secreted sooner after you eat, which makes it work more efficiently. GLP-1 also acts on the brain to forestall hunger.

It turns out that the GLP-1 of most people who are obese or have diabetes is underactive. That's where GLP-1 *analogs* come in. Synthetic versions of the natural hormone, they perform all of the actions of GLP-1. As with natural GLP-1, the analogs affect several aspects of carbohydrate processing rather than just one, as metformin and acarbose do. Restoring GLP-1 function with GLP-1 analogs not only improves blood sugar, cholesterol balance, and blood pressure but also causes significant, sometimes dramatic, weight loss, especially when combined with metformin. In a study reported in the journal *Diabetes, Obesity and Metabolism* by Ochsner Health System researchers in New Orleans, obese subjects with type 2 diabetes who used the GLP-1 analog exenatide lost an average of 16 pounds and were still losing weight when the study ended after a year and a half. No weight loss drug has ever come close to matching those results. Remarkably, these subjects weren't taking the medication to lose weight; they were mainly interested in treating their diabetes.

The two GLP-1 analogs currently available are exenatide (pharmaceutical name: Byetta) and liraglutide (pharmaceutical name: Victoza). Both are taken by self-injection. They come in convenient "pens" that can be carried in your pocket like a writing pen. The needles are only about $^1/_4$ inch long and are so thin that people rarely complain of discomfort when injecting. Only a few drops of the medication are required each day.

Exenatide is usually taken twice a day before meals; liraglutide is taken once a day without regard to meals. The only common side effect is nausea, which usually subsides in a few days. Serious side effects are unusual. There have been reports of pancreatitis—inflammation of the pancreas— but this has been rare and resolved quickly after the patients stopped taking the medication.

A similar medication, pramlintide (pharmaceutical name: Symlin), works the way GLP-1 analogs do. It slows stomach emptying, helps the liver remove glucose from the bloodstream after meals, and reduces after-meal glucose levels. Like other sugar blockers, it reduces blood sugar and insulin demands. As with the GLP-1 analogs, it's self-administered with a pen-type injector. Doctors sometimes prescribe pramlintide in place of mealtime insulin injections to reduce after-meal glucose spikes. Unlike mealtime insulin injections, which cause weight gain, pramlintide promotes mild weight loss, although not as much as the GLP-1 analogs.

Another class of medications, called gliptins, raise levels of your own GLP-1 by inhibiting the enzyme that breaks down GLP-1. These include sitagliptin (pharmaceutical name: Januvia) and saxagliptin (pharmaceutical name: Onglyza). Like GLP-1 analogs, gliptins improve after-meal blood sugar levels and overall diabetes control without causing weight gain. However, they don't cause much weight loss. The main advantage of gliptins over GLP-1 analogs is that they're taken as pills instead of injections.

The reason GLP-1 analogs are so effective at causing weight loss may stem from the fact that they block sugar at several points in the digestive process, not just one. As you learned in the discussion of sugar-blocking foods, combinations of foods that act on different parts of your digestive system to block sugar work better than ones that act on only one. GLP-1 analogs—which slow stomach emptying, help the liver absorb glucose,

TZDs: RECENT QUESTIONS ABOUT SAFETY

ROSIGLITAZONE (Avandia) and pioglitazone (Actos) belong to a unique class of insulin-sensitizing medications called thiazolidinediones, or TZDs. These drugs are effective for lowering blood sugar and insulin levels, and have been found to slow the loss of insulin-producing beta cells. However, they sometimes have undesirable side effects. Instead of promoting weight loss, as other insulin-sensitizing drugs do, they actually encourage mild weight gain. They also cause fluid retention, which can be dangerous in some patients with heart disease.

The FDA recently prohibited the sale of rosiglitazone because some studies showed an increased rate of heart attacks among patients using it. No such risk has been found with pioglitazone.

and enhance first-phase insulin secretion all at once—work better than metformin or acarbose, which affect only one part of the digestive process. Several studies have shown that combining exenatide with metformin produces significantly more weight loss than using exenatide alone.

● DIET PLUS SUGAR-BLOCKING MEDICATIONS: A POWERFUL COMBINATION

If you're, say, 50 pounds overweight, losing 16 pounds—the amount of weight loss produced by exenatide in the study mentioned above— would certainly be welcome, but undoubtedly you would like to lose more. As the Saint Louis University study mentioned above showed, insulin sensitizers are especially effective when combined with a good weight loss program. If you combined regular exercise of your slow-twitch muscle fibers, a low–glycemic load diet, natural sugar blockers, and medicinal sugar blockers, you would optimize not only the beneficial effects of sugar blocking on your blood sugar and insulin levels but also your chances of attaining a healthy body weight.

Of course, the idea of staying on a medication for the rest of your life probably doesn't appeal to you. However, you can look upon medications as a bridge to a better lifestyle. Weight loss by any means improves insulin sensitivity and can initiate a virtuous cycle. Restoring insulin sensitivity promotes weight loss, which in turn increases insulin sensitivity. Even if you stop taking the medication, your body won't need as much insulin as it did before. Lower insulin levels will help relieve the internal starvation that causes you to be overly hungry. Also, when you lose weight by any means, exercising becomes easier, which improves insulin sensitivity and encourages even more weight loss. If taking the medications results in positive changes in your lifestyle, chances are there will be no need to continue taking the drug.

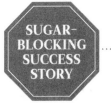
Age: 38

Height: 5' 3"

Pounds lost: 8½

Inches lost: 12¾

Major accomplishments: Learning to adapt to proper eating habits and starting a regular exercise routine.

Favorite sugar blockers: Pickles!

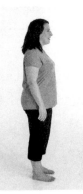

before

RENEE MARCHISOTTO

A Cure for the Common Crankiness

DURING PREGNANCY, Renee Marchisotto experienced gestational diabetes, a form of the disease that occurs only during pregnancy. "Having gestational diabetes was quite a surprise to me, and unfortunately I was one of the small percentage of expectant mothers who had to take insulin via injection, as well as [be on] a very controlled, restrictive diet," said Renee. "I was told by my obstetrician and my endocrinologist that [because of this] I was at a higher risk for developing type 2 diabetes."

Renee had other factors pushing her toward the Sugar Blockers Diet—her weight and polycystic ovary syndrome also put her at risk.

She had had some success with other weight loss plans but found it more and more difficult to stick with them afterward. Between work and motherhood, carving out time to exercise seemed harder each day. But as her daughter grew more active (she's now 3), Renee wanted to grow more active with her.

"I wanted to be able to keep up with my daughter physically, especially as she gets older. I love the outdoors and want to be able to share this with her, without any limitations due to my lack of physical agility," she said. Soon after, Renee started the Sugar Blockers Diet—and 6 weeks later was well on her way to achieving that goal, having lost 8 pounds and more than 12 inches.

How'd she do it? "I really enjoy exercising. I had missed it . . . and now I make sure it's a priority," says

Renee, who would even host impromptu Pilates classes at work in empty offices. "If I didn't take a break away from my desk to get out and walk or do something, I didn't have as clear a head, I wasn't as refreshed, and the afternoons seemed longer." And she's not the only one who saw the difference that movement made in her day: "My boss would even tell me to go for my walk or go do what I need to do because he noticed I would come back feeling better," she said. "If I don't exercise or walk, I'm cranky."

Renee also recognized how certain foods affect her moods and how diet and exercise are linked through more than just weight. "I'm much more conscious of what I eat now. My saving grace was $1/2$ cup of very dark, very rich chocolate ice cream." Just a taste was all she needed to keep her happy, and too many sweets, especially processed ones, could actually result in some midday grouchiness.

"I feel really well," Renee said, beaming. "This has been a life-changing experience for me."

She is now more than equipped with the food and exercise knowledge she needs (in fact, the program spurred her to permanently keep an eye on her blood sugar and to make more regular doctor's appointments) to keep her energy level on a par with that of her toddler daughter. And as an added benefit, she lost a dress size: "It's nice to be able to fit back into clothes I fit into pre-pregnancy!"

after

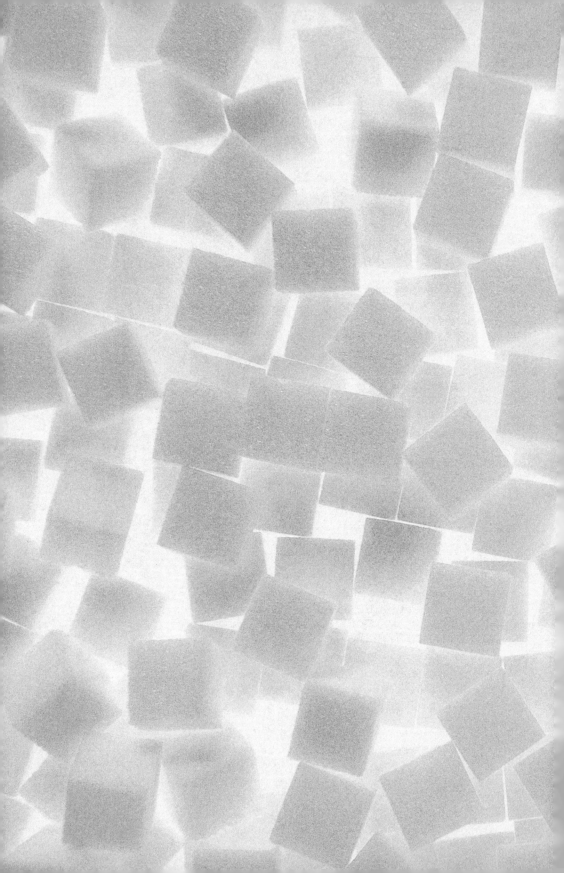

14

BLOCKING SUGAR'S EFFECTS ON **YOUR** ARTERIES

"YOU'RE ONLY AS OLD as your arteries." Those words, made famous by Dr. William Osler (1849–1919), the "Father of Modern Medicine," are as true now as they were in his day. Most of us live only as long as our arteries let us. Cardiovascular disease causes more deaths than all other diseases combined.

Look at it this way: Every cell in your body is surrounded by a membrane that controls what goes in and out of it. These walls protect cells from potentially harmful substances in the blood, including high blood sugar. Cell membranes are, in essence, the ultimate sugar blocker. No matter how much sugar you have in your blood, it can't get into your cells unless they need it.

It's a different story for the pipes that carry blood to your cells—your arteries. They're exposed to everything in your bloodstream, including high blood sugar, high levels of bad cholesterol, insufficient levels of good cholesterol, and carbon monoxide from cigarette smoking. In addition, your arteries have to absorb the pressure pulsations generated by your heart pumping blood through your system. Consequently, high blood sugar, high blood cholesterol, low levels of good cholesterol, high blood pressure, and cigarette smoking all damage your arteries.

You can use the sugar blockers discussed in this book to keep excessive sugar from rushing into your bloodstream. The cell membranes block excessive sugar from going into your cells. However, there's no blocker between the sugar in your blood and the walls of your arteries. They're directly exposed. That's why diabetes is essentially a disease of the arteries. Artery damage is what causes the eye and kidney problems that diabetics get, as well as heart attacks and strokes. If you can keep your blood vessels healthy, you are unlikely to suffer any ill effects from diabetes.

Here's how you can "block" the effects of high blood sugar on your arteries.

● PAY ATTENTION TO FOUR NUMBERS

If you've ever bought life insurance, you might remember somebody measuring your blood pressure, taking a blood sample, and asking you if you smoke. Insurance companies place bets on how long your arteries will last, and the best way to estimate that is to measure your blood pressure, blood sugar, and good and bad cholesterol levels, and to find out if you use tobacco.

Actually, arteries are remarkably tough. They're resistant to infection and cancer. The only disease that commonly affects arteries is atherosclerosis, damage from the infiltration and buildup of cholesterol. Every doctor knows the four major risk factors for atherosclerosis:

- High blood cholesterol
- High blood pressure
- Diabetes
- Cigarette smoking

The more of those risk factors you have, and the further from normal each is, the greater your risk.

Risk factors "potentiate" one another—that is, each makes the others more potent. For example, whereas high blood cholesterol might double your risk of heart disease, if you're diabetic, the same degree of high cholesterol could quadruple your risk. In other words, having two risk factors is not just a little worse than having one—it's much worse.

Here's the good news: This also works in reverse. Having only one risk factor isn't just a little better than having two—it's a lot better. Actually, many of us eventually come up with one of those four risk factors, but most of us don't develop artery problems, at least until we're very old. Most heart attacks and strokes occur in people who have more than one major risk factor for atherosclerosis.

Of course, the best of all worlds would be to have no risk factors. Nevertheless, type 2 diabetes *alone* doesn't cause much trouble if you don't have any other risk factors—if your cholesterol and blood pressure levels are normal and you don't smoke. However, if you have diabetes, it becomes especially important not to have any other risk factors. Taking care of your arteries is not about just one number, your blood sugar level. It's about four numbers: your blood sugar, cholesterol, blood pressure, and how many cigarettes you smoke.

"Better Than Normal"

Here's a common scenario: Joe has always been pleased with his blood cholesterol level. It's always been normal. However, when he developed type 2 diabetes, his doctor told him that, in addition to medication for diabetes, he would need to take cholesterol-lowering pills. Why would Joe have to take medication for his cholesterol if it was normal to begin with?

If you have diabetes, a "normal" cholesterol level isn't necessarily the best cholesterol. Ideally, it should be lower than normal. Here's why: Just as risk factors can add to one another, they can also *subtract* from one another. Having a cholesterol level that is lower than normal makes up for some of the risk of having blood sugar that is higher than normal.

But isn't it best to be normal? In medicine, "normal" usually just means *average*. However, average isn't necessarily ideal. For example, the average American's weight is high enough to increase his or her risk of diabetes and heart disease. Thus, it's healthier to weigh less than average. The same is true of cholesterol and blood pressure. It's better to have cholesterol and blood pressure levels that are lower than average. Indeed, people with lower-than-average cholesterol levels and blood pressure live longer than average. This is especially true if you have diabetes, because diabetes makes blood vessels extra sensitive to the damaging effects of high blood cholesterol, high blood pressure, and smoking. Lowering your cholesterol and blood pressure to below-average levels—and, of course, quitting smoking—offsets much of the risk of having high blood sugar.

As far as medical science knows, there's no downside to having a lower-than-average cholesterol level—the lower the better. Experts recommend that people with diabetes keep their bad-cholesterol levels well below average, which is why Joe's doctor told him to take cholesterol-lowering medication even though his cholesterol level was "normal."

Similarly, diabetes organizations recommend that people with diabetes be particularly vigilant about treating high blood pressure. However, there are downsides to having blood pressure that's too low. You need enough pressure in your arteries to pump blood to your brain. If your blood pressure gets too low, you could faint. Also, recent evidence suggests that, while correcting high blood pressure reduces the risk of heart attacks and strokes, having excessively low blood pressure can actually increase the risk of heart attack. Experts are currently debating how low your blood pressure should be if you have diabetes. Until they figure it out, you should be especially careful to keep it at least at levels considered acceptable for nondiabetics.

● LOWERING YOUR CHOLESTEROL

When doctors check cholesterol these days, they measure LDL, or bad cholesterol, and HDL, or good cholesterol. When they talk about lowering blood cholesterol, they usually mean the bad-cholesterol level. The lower your LDL level, the lower your risk of artery problems, including heart attack and stroke.

While type 2 diabetes is all about diet and exercise, your bad-cholesterol level is a different matter. As discussed in Chapter 5, contrary to popular conception, high blood cholesterol is not caused by eating fat and cholesterol. LDL levels really don't change much with diet and exercise.

Back in the 1960s, when researchers discovered a relationship between high blood cholesterol and heart attacks, the idea that high blood cholesterol came from eating too much fat and cholesterol sounded reasonable to some scientists, but that notion turned out to be an oversimplification. Your liver makes most of the cholesterol in your blood—about three times more than comes from food. If you eat less cholesterol, your liver just makes more; if you eat more, it makes less.

Cholesterol is a vital substance. You couldn't live 5 minutes without it. Your body needs cholesterol to build cell membranes, hormones, and other important things. Mother Nature wasn't foolish enough to rely on the vagaries of food intake to supply our bodies with cholesterol.

Cholesterol is actually difficult to absorb from food. Most of the cholesterol you eat passes right out in your stool. This is particularly true if you are overweight or have type 2 diabetes, in which case your liver often produces more cholesterol particles than normal (see Chapter 2) and your intestines compensate by absorbing less than normal.

The level of bad cholesterol in your blood depends not on how much cholesterol goes into your body but rather on how much of it your body chooses to let out, and that's based mainly on genetics. Indeed, scientists have discovered more than 1,600 different genetic quirks that raise LDL. The human gene pool is full of them. About a third of the human population has some kind of genetic quirk in their cholesterol metabolism.

Why did Mother Nature do this to us? High blood cholesterol rarely causes trouble before age 40. For millions of years, humans didn't live long enough to be affected by high blood cholesterol—the average life span was less than 40 years. Consequently, genetic quirks in cholesterol metabolism accumulated harmlessly in the gene pool. Only in the past few hundred years, as people began living longer, has high blood cholesterol influenced survival. Now these quirks influence how long many of us live.

Considering that genes, rather than lifestyle, determine your bad-cholesterol level, it's not surprising that diet and exercise usually don't influence it much. However, you've probably heard of people going on strict diets and lowering their cholesterol levels. Several things happen when you change your diet and exercise habits that can make you *think* you've succeeded in lowering your bad-cholesterol level when you really haven't. If you lose weight by any means, your cholesterol level will often fall while you're losing it but will usually come right back up when you stabilize at a new weight. The opposite is also true. When you gain weight, your cholesterol level will rise as you are gaining but go back down after you stop.

In the Dietary Modification Trial of the Women's Health Initiative, discussed in Chapter 5, researchers examined the effects of a low-fat, low-cholesterol diet on cholesterol levels and on the incidence of heart disease in more than 18,000 American women. These women underwent an intense training program to teach them to reduce fat and cholesterol in their diets. It did no good: After 8 years, bad-cholesterol levels fell on average by less than 2 percent, and there was no reduction in the incidence of heart disease.

If you're overweight or have type 2 diabetes or prediabetes, there's a significant downside to low-fat, low-cholesterol diets. If you cut out eggs, meat, and dairy products, you're bound to increase your intake of refined carbohydrates—the last thing you need.

What about exercise? It's great for losing weight, lowering blood sugar, and preventing diabetes. It also raises good-cholesterol levels. However, it doesn't lower bad-cholesterol levels.

If diet and exercise don't work, how can you lower your LDL level? The most effective way to lower bad-cholesterol levels is to take cholesterol-lowering medication. Here's how it works.

Your liver cells have tiny receptors on their surfaces that pull bad cholesterol out of your blood and into the cells, where it can be broken down and eliminated. The reason some people's LDL levels are higher than others' is that those receptors are genetically less active.

In the 1980s, a couple of American scientists won a Nobel Prize for deciphering the enzyme system that controls the number of receptors in liver cells. Pharmaceutical companies came up with a type of medication derived from natural cholesterol-lowering substances in yeast. They are called statins, and they lower cholesterol by boosting the numbers of LDL receptors in liver cells.

These cholesterol-lowering medications have been one of the seminal achievements of modern medicine. One pill a day can reduce bad-cholesterol

LDL Cholesterol:
HOW LOW IS IDEAL FOR YOU?

THE AVERAGE LDL in the United States is approximately 140. According to the National Institutes of Health guidelines used by most specialists, if you have no other risk factors—cigarette smoking, high blood pressure, low levels of good cholesterol, or a family history of heart disease—your LDL is okay as long as it is less than 160. If you have one or more of those risk factors, the guidelines suggest lowering it to 130 or less. If you already have narrow or blocked arteries, it should be less than 100. Because diabetes makes your arteries vulnerable to the damaging effects of cholesterol, the guidelines recommend that if you have diabetes, you should keep your LDL below 100, whether or not you have other risk factors.

levels by more than 50 percent. Thanks to these medications, the incidence of heart attacks in the United States has plummeted.

If you're taking a statin, you don't need to worry about eating fat and cholesterol. It won't raise your bad-cholesterol level a bit. Just to be sure, researchers reporting their results in the journal *Mayo Clinic Proceedings* put patients taking statins on an extremely high-fat diet for 6 weeks. Participants avoided starch but ate *a pound and a half* of meat and cheese a day. At the end of the study, the patients' blood sugar and insulin levels dropped, and they lost an average of 12 pounds. The balance between their good and bad cholesterol levels looked better than ever. On average, their good-cholesterol levels went up, and their bad-cholesterol levels stayed the same.

Remember, it's not how much cholesterol is going into your body that determines your cholesterol level; it's how much your liver chooses to let out, and that's controlled by a genetic "set point"—like a thermostat. Statins lower the setting on that thermostat.

Statins are safer than aspirin. The only common side effect is muscle soreness, which affects approximately 1 in 10 people who take them. You can sometimes avoid this by reducing the statin dose and adding other medications to boost the statin's cholesterol-lowering effects. Serious side effects are rare. The most dangerous one is diffuse muscle damage, which can injure the kidneys.

● RAISING YOUR GOOD CHOLESTEROL

The reason you may want to lower your bad cholesterol is clear enough. Cholesterol builds up in your arteries and blocks them off. It makes sense to keep the levels down. However, the concept of good cholesterol is harder to grasp. How can cholesterol be good if it damages your arteries?

Your good-cholesterol level is a measure of the amount of cholesterol in particles called high-density lipoproteins (HDL). The more of these particles you have, the better off you are. However, it's not actually the cholesterol in HDL particles that provides benefit; it's the other parts of the particles that do the work. These particles contain a host of complex proteins that perform many beneficial functions. In addition to removing cholesterol from the walls of arteries, they reduce inflammation, prevent blood clots, fight infection, and suppress tumor growth. The bottom line: It's good to have lots of HDL. A 1 percent increase in your HDL level lowers your risk of heart disease by as much as a 3 percent decrease in your bad-cholesterol level does.

When patients ask doctors how they can raise their HDL levels, they're often told that there isn't much they can do, other than lowering their bad cholesterol to offset the effects of not having enough good cholesterol. Exercise helps a little. So does moderate alcohol intake. But patients usually end

WHAT SHOULD YOUR HDL Level BE?

THE AVERAGE HDL level in the United States is around 45 for men and 55 for women. Generally, the higher your HDL level, the lower your risk of heart and blood vessel disease. The National Institutes of Health guidelines consider HDL levels lower than 40 to be a significant risk factor and levels greater than 60 to be partially protective. Of course, your risk also depends on how high your bad-cholesterol (LDL) level is. As it turns out, the most accurate predictor is the ratio between the total amount of cholesterol in your blood and your good-cholesterol level—your

cholesterol-to-HDL ratio. For example, if your total cholesterol level is 200 and your HDL level is 50, your cholesterol-to-HDL ratio would be 4.0.

The average cholesterol-to-HDL ratio in the United States is approximately 4.5. A ratio greater than 6 would be considered a significant risk factor. If you have other risk factors for blood vessel disease besides cholesterol imbalance—such as diabetes, high blood pressure, cigarette smoking, or a family history of premature blood vessel disease— many specialists recommend getting your ratio below 3.0.

up with the impression that, while they can lower their bad-cholesterol levels with diet and exercise, their good-cholesterol level is largely unchangeable.

Ironically, *it's the exact opposite.* It's your bad-cholesterol level that is largely unchanged by diet and exercise. Your HDL is highly dependent on your lifestyle and significantly influenced by diet and exercise. How did this get overlooked? Until recently, doctors recommended low-fat, low-cholesterol diets for cholesterol problems, which actually *lower HDL levels.* It's no wonder that doctors thought diet and exercise did no good: The kinds of diets they were prescribing actually made the problem worse.

Here's the good news: While low-fat diets lower HDL levels, low-*carbohydrate* diets raise them.

In fact, scientists have known for years that low-carbohydrate diets raise good cholesterol *slightly*—by approximately 5 percent. They have also known for years that exercise raises HDL levels *slightly*—again, by about 5 percent. But what if you exercise *and* cut carbs? Only recently have researchers carefully studied what happens when you do both. University of Pennsylvania researchers randomly divided 307 subjects into two groups. They gave one group the usual advice to avoid fat and cholesterol and count calories, without giving them specific instructions to exercise. They told the other group to avoid carbohydrates and walk 50 minutes five times a week. The group that cut carbs and exercised increased their HDL levels by 23 percent more than the subjects who didn't exercise—results that match any medication available today.

Most people who have low levels of HDL (less than 40 for men, less than 50 for women) have high blood triglyceride levels. As you'll recall, your liver converts excess carbs to triglycerides and sends them through your bloodstream to be stored as fat. Although triglyceride itself is largely harmless, high levels of it "wash away" good cholesterol. If you cut out carbs and exercise regularly, after a few days your triglyceride levels will drop, and after a few weeks your HDL levels will usually rise. Losing

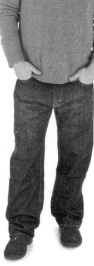

JEREMY GIANDOMENICO

IF YOU HAD SEEN A PHOTOGRAPH of Jeremy Giandomenico prior to his joining the Sugar Blockers Diet, you would have thought: "Why is this seemingly fit young man starting a weight loss program?"

But 5 years prior, at age 30, Jeremy was diagnosed as prediabetic. Because his father had type 2 diabetes and heart disease, Jeremy knew what that meant for his own health, and yet he hadn't been able to find a way to improve his risk factors. Even though he worked out 5 days a week, when he started the Sugar Blockers Diet his cholesterol and triglyceride levels were so high that they were literally off the charts. "When I found out how bad my numbers were, I felt like a freight train hit me," said Jeremy. "I was devastated to see how bad [they] were."

Jeremy's mother, Joan, had also joined the Sugar Blockers Diet and was working toward getting her own blood sugar lowered, as well as the number she saw on the scale. "My husband has had a heart attack and has diabetes," said Joan. "And Jeremy follows in his father's footsteps. I'm happy to see he's trying to keep his numbers under control so maybe that won't happen to him, too."

After just 6 weeks on the Sugar Blockers Diet, Jeremy

Age: 35
Lost 7½ pounds
and 6" in 6 weeks

weight, quitting smoking, and moderating alcohol consumption all add to the HDL-raising effects of cutting carbs and exercising. Indeed, lifestyle changes can raise HDL levels by as much as 50 percent.

was amazed by his progress—and so was his family. His fasting blood sugar levels, which were 381 at the beginning of the program (high enough for him to be considered diabetic), came down a whopping 205 points, while his triglyceride level improved by more than 500—by far the biggest drop in numbers across the board when it came to our test panelists. His doctor, Jeremy reported, was "very impressed with the test results I showed him."

And he did it all with food, no drugs! Said Jeremy, "I was not on any medication during the program. I wanted to see how much of an effect the Sugar Blockers Diet would have before I went to my doctor, and I was amazed by how much difference just changing my eating habits had."

Motivated to make a change for his better health, Jeremy not only continued to eat and exercise the Sugar Blockers Diet way but also started a short course of blood pressure and cholesterol-lowering medications. Four months after the program ended, his triglyceride level—which had started at greater than 650 (more than the instrument measures)—was an amazing 66 and his total cholesterol level less than 100. His blood pressure and blood sugar levels also improved.

Jeremy noted, "It has been pretty easy to stick with this program. I still plan to try and lower my numbers even more and lose more weight. As long as I stick to this program, I know it will keep working."

There is a small minority of people with low levels of good cholesterol for whom diet and exercise do not work. Most of these individuals have a genetic quirk in their HDL metabolism that keeps their good-cholesterol levels low no matter how hard they work at it. It is possible to recognize such people by measuring their triglyceride levels. If those levels are always normal (less than 125), diet and exercise are unlikely to raise HDL.

To increase HDL, doctors sometimes prescribe the vitamin niacin in much larger doses than needed to avoid deficiency. Niacin raises HDL and has been proven to reduce the risk of heart disease. The problem with niacin is that it often causes annoying flushing and hot flashes. Although these usually subside after a few months of taking the drug, they often discourage people from staying on it.

Another HDL-raising medication is a type of drug called a fibrate. It's relatively free of side effects, but studies of the drug's effectiveness have been inconsistent. It does reduce the risk of heart disease in people with high triglyceride levels (more than 200) combined with low HDL levels (less than 40)—the same people who are able to raise their HDL levels by cutting carbs and exercising.

● LOWERING YOUR BLOOD PRESSURE

Insulin resistance and diabetes increase your chances of developing high blood pressure. In turn, high blood pressure adds to the damaging effects on your arteries of insulin resistance and diabetes. You can reduce your risk of artery damage by taking measures to keep your blood pressure down.

The pressure in your arteries rises and falls with each beat of your heart. The peak to which your pressure rises with each beat is called the systolic blood pressure; the depth to which it falls between beats is the diastolic blood pressure. Normal blood pressure for young adults is less than 120 for the systolic and less than 80 for the diastolic, expressed as 120/80.

For nondiabetics, the National Institutes of Health (NIH) recommends treatment to keep blood pressure 140/90 or less. However, for diabetics, some professional organizations recommend 130/80 or less, although this is controversial. If getting your blood pressure that low requires only one or two medications, then it appears to be beneficial. However, if you need more than that, the downsides of trying to get it that low begin to outweigh the benefits, in which case 140/90 is sufficient.

Sometimes it's hard to figure out whether you have high blood pressure or not. Blood pressure fluctuates from day to day, hour to hour, even from minute to minute. If your blood pressure is high every time you check it, you can reasonably conclude that you have high blood pressure. However, it may be high at times and low at others. Even people who don't have harmful high blood pressure have occasional high readings when they're nervous or excited.

As you get older, your arteries normally get stiffer, and that raises your systolic blood pressure. If you live long enough, chances are it will exceed 140, the point at which the NIH guidelines recommend treatment. In other words, the guidelines suggest treating something that occurs naturally in most people. As common as this age-related rise is, it still increases the wear and tear on your arteries. Research has shown that, regardless of your age, if you can keep your systolic blood pressure below 140, you will reduce your risk of stroke and heart disease.

The increased artery stiffness that occurs with age also causes your systolic blood pressure to fluctuate more. Before concluding that you need additional medication, you should get several readings spaced at least a week apart to make sure that your blood pressure is consistently high.

If blood pressure is only a few points higher than normal, doctors often recommend trying some lifestyle changes first. Reducing sodium helps a little, as does increasing your intake of potassium, which you get in fruits

High Blood Pressure:
ECHOES OF A SALT-SCARCE PAST

THESE DAYS salt is cheap and widely available, but it wasn't always so easy to get. In prehistoric times, humans often suffered from *lack* of salt. Indeed, their ability to go without food and water for long periods depended in large part on the amount of salt in their bodies.

One of your kidney's main jobs is to pull salt molecules from the urine and put them back into your bloodstream. It's a survival mechanism. Your ability to withstand dehydration depends largely on your kidneys' ability to retrieve salt. This requires work on the part of your kidneys. The healthier your kidneys are, the better they are at preventing salt from leaving the body.

You could say that high blood pressure is an echo of our salt-scarce past. Our kidneys evolved to be more efficient at retrieving salt than we need them to be. Many people's kidneys are overly reluctant to release salt into the urine, which triggers reflexes that raise blood pressure. Indeed, for most people, high blood pressure can be easily treated with a mild diuretic, which lets the kidneys release salt.

Avoiding salt in the diet doesn't work very well for lowering blood pressure because the amount of salt in your body depends little on how much salt is going into your system. It's more a matter of how much your kidneys let out.

Most people's blood pressures rise as they age. It's hard to call high blood pressure a disease when it's actually the manifestation of a survival mechanism that was once invaluable but is no longer needed. Nevertheless, it increases the risk of blood vessel disease, and treating it prevents heart attacks and strokes.

and vegetables. Research shows that cutting carbs helps. Cutting fat and cholesterol has no effect.

The reality, though, is that high blood pressure is difficult to control with diet and exercise alone. If lifestyle changes don't bring your blood pressure down, you should not hesitate to take medication to lower it. The longer you let high blood pressure go untreated, the harder it is to control it. The good news is that one or two pills a day will usually lower your blood pressure to where it should be.

A word of caution: Lowering your *systolic* blood pressure when your *diastolic* pressure is normal can be tricky. It's important to try to get the systolic pressure under 140, but medication that's too strong can cause an unsafe drop in blood pressure in this situation.

● TOO MANY NUMBERS? LOOK AT THE BRIGHT SIDE

Taking care of your blood vessels is not just about one number—your blood sugar, cholesterol, blood pressure, cigarette smoking—it's about all four. Reducing sugar shocks with the Sugar Blockers Diet not only will lower your blood sugar but also will improve the balance between your good- and bad-cholesterol levels and even help lower your blood pressure. And if diet, exercise, and other lifestyle changes aren't enough, be thankful that we have medications that really work. The bottom line is, if you keep those numbers where they should be, you can live to a ripe old age without missing a day of active living because of blood vessel problems, heart disease, or diabetes.

CONCLUSION

---•

B
EFORE READING this book, you might have thought that the only means you had for losing weight or controlling your blood sugar was to go on a strict diet or engage in strenuous exercise. By considering the physiological causes of obesity and type 2 diabetes, you've learned that the driving force behind diabesity is excessive demands for insulin caused by insulin resistance and excessive starch consumption. Refined carbohydrates increase insulin demands largely by causing after-meal blood sugar spikes. The key to losing weight and preventing or treating type 2 diabetes is not just to cut carbs but to reduce after-meal blood sugar spikes by using sugar blockers. It's also important to target physical activity toward restoring your body's sensitivity to insulin.

Australian researchers recently reported in the *American Journal of Clinical Nutrition* that, in people going about their usual activities, it was difficult to predict their blood sugar or insulin responses to typical meals just by measuring the carbohydrate content of the foods they ate. Only when the researchers took into consideration the glycemic load of the foods were they able to predict after-meal blood sugar and insulin levels with any degree of accuracy. However, while the glycemic load was 85 percent accurate in predicting after-meal blood sugar responses to *single* foods, it explained only 58 percent of the difference in after-meal levels among people eating *mixed* meals during a normal day. Such factors as interactions between foods, the order in which foods are consumed, activities before and after eating, stress, and the quality of sleep cause variations in the way the body handles carbohydrates. Although those elements make predicting blood sugar responses more difficult, there's potential here for a new tool in combating both obesity and diabetes: sugar blockers.

As you have seen, you can use knowledge of these effects to blunt after-meal blood sugar spikes, the driver of excessive insulin production. Sugar-blocking substances in foods like fiber-rich fruits and vegetables, fatty nuts and seeds, and protein-rich meats all help slow down the digestion of starches to soften sugar shocks. In addition, other sugar-blocking strategies, such as taking a brisk walk after eating and relaxing at mealtimes, can help you avoid postmeal surges. Indeed, the starch-blocking medication acarbose taught us that it takes only a little reduction in after-meal blood sugar levels to curb insulin demands, improve cholesterol balance, lower blood pressure, and reduce the risk of diabetes.

Finally, remember that you're only as old as your arteries and that the health of your blood vessels depends not just on one number—your blood sugar, cholesterol, blood pressure, or cigarette smoking—but on all four. Living the Sugar Blockers Diet way is an easy and delicious way to improve your numbers, as several of our test panelists did. So eat up and enjoy a long, healthy life of sugar blocking!

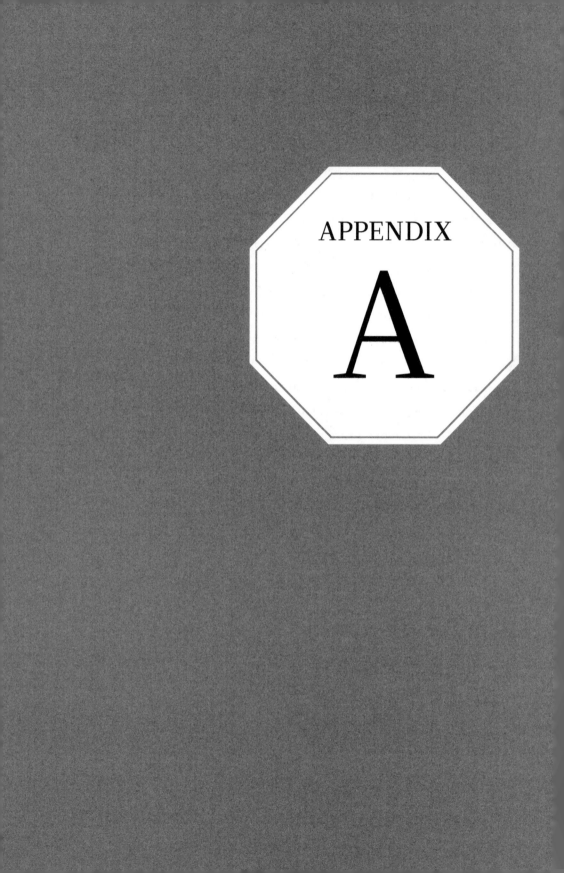

APPENDIX

A

SUGAR BLOCKERS
DIET MENUS

THE FOLLOWING 2 WEEKS of menus are an example of how to eat the Sugar Blockers Diet way. See how easy it is to eat heartily while abiding by the rule of no more than the equivalent of one full serving of starch per day and no sugar-containing beverages. These menus incorporate some of the delicious recipes from Chapter 9 and give you ideas on how to throw together some quick and easy meals, but they also allow you to eat out if you choose. Having a daily pattern—in this case, light breakfasts and lunches, larger dinners, and only occasional snacks—helps prevent random eating.

Notice in these menus that starch is almost always consumed with protein, frequently preceded by a fatty appetizer to slow stomach emptying, and accompanied by a hearty salad and a serving of vegetables to raise the fiber content to approximately 10 grams. Other sugar blockers—such as vinegar, olive oil, alcohol, chia seeds, and (in rare instances) acarbose—further lower the glycemic load. Sweets are eaten only after meals.

MONDAY

●

BREAKFAST

Coffee, tea, tomato juice, or milk

2-egg omelet with cheese, mushrooms, and bacon

Apple slices

LUNCH

Coffee, tea, milk, or water

Classic Cobb Salad (see page 165)

1 slice of bread, consumed after half of the salad is eaten

DINNER

APPETIZER: cheese

Red wine, milk, or water

SALAD: romaine lettuce, assorted vegetables, and nuts
with dressing: vinegar and olive oil

Steak shish kebab with green peppers, mushrooms,
zucchini, and onion

1 baked potato skin with sour cream and butter

DESSERT: grapes

Coffee or tea

TUESDAY

●

BREAKFAST

Coffee, tea, tomato juice, or milk

1 Berry Wrap (see page 157)

LUNCH

Milk or water

STARTER SALAD: lettuce, tomato, olives, and walnuts
with dressing: vinegar and olive oil

Grilled halibut

Green vegetable

½ cup rice

Coffee or tea

DINNER

APPETIZER: peanuts

White wine, milk, or water

SALAD: spinach, bacon bits, Parmesan cheese,
and walnuts with dressing: vinegar and olive oil

Chicken Cacciatore (see page 193)

Broccoli

1 cup fettuccine

DESSERT: 2 clusters chocolate-covered nuts

Coffee or tea

WEDNESDAY

●

BREAKFAST

Coffee, tea, tomato juice, or milk

Orange slices

Eggs Rancheros (see page 153)

1 slice of toast with butter

LUNCH

Diet soda, milk, or water

French onion soup

Turkey, Swiss cheese, avocado, and tomato wrap

Coffee, tea, or milk

SNACK

Almonds

DINNER

White wine, beer, milk, or water

Caesar salad

Baked salmon

Spinach sprinkled with vinegar

Fauxtatoes (see page 201)

DESSERT: 6 hot-cinnamon jelly beans

Coffee or tea

THURSDAY

●

BREAKFAST

Coffee, tea, tomato juice, or milk

½ cup bran cereal with 3 tablespoons chopped walnuts

2 microwaved eggs

LUNCH

Diet soda, milk, or water

Teriyaki stir-fried chicken and vegetables

½ cup rice

Coffee or tea

DINNER

APPETIZER: Cajun Nut Mix (see page 176)

Red wine, diet soda, or milk

SALAD: iceberg lettuce, tomato,
and bacon bits with blue cheese dressing and
sprinkled with vinegar

3 slices Italian sausage pizza (cut away two-thirds of crust)

DESSERT: dark chocolate

Coffee or tea

FRIDAY

●

BREAKFAST

Coffee, tea, tomato juice, or milk

½ grapefruit

1 bowl equal parts unsweetened yogurt, berries,
and All-Bran cereal with 2 tablespoons chia seeds

LUNCH

Beer, diet soda, milk, or water

Beef chili

Coffee or tea

DINNER

100 mg acarbose, taken immediately before eating

APPETIZER: Caprese salad (mozzarella cheese,
tomato, basil, and olive oil)

Red wine, water, or milk

SALAD: romaine lettuce, walnuts, feta cheese,
red peppers, and tomato

1 cup spaghetti with 1 cup meat sauce

Steamed spinach, butter, and lemon juice

DESSERT: dark chocolate

Coffee or tea

SATURDAY

●

BREAKFAST

Coffee, tea, tomato juice, or milk

2 slices of bacon

2 eggs, any style

1 slice of Green Banana–Nut Bread (see page 159)

LUNCH

Beer, diet soda, milk, or water

Green salad with dressing: vinegar and olive oil

Deluxe cheeseburger with top bun removed

Coffee or tea

DINNER

APPETIZER: mixed nuts

Red wine, milk, or water

SALAD: lettuce, nuts, and chunks of assorted
vegetables with dressing: equal parts vinegar and olive oil
and blue cheese

Sausage and Peppers (see page 196)

Asparagus

$\frac{1}{2}$ cup garlic mashed potatoes

DESSERT: yogurt and raspberries sweetened
with $\frac{1}{2}$ teaspoon sugar

Coffee or tea

SUNDAY

●

BREAKFAST

Coffee, tea, or milk

Raspberries topped with milk or cream

Scrambled Eggs with Pesto and Ricotta (see page 152)

1 slice of toast with butter and 1 teaspoon jam

LUNCH

Diet soda, milk, or water

Roast beef wrap with low-carb tortilla

Apple slices

Coffee or tea

SNACK

Pork rinds

DINNER

Beer, red wine, milk, or water

SALAD: Bibb lettuce, nuts, and assorted vegetables
with ranch dressing

Barbecued chicken

Collard greens

Fruit salad

DESSERT: 2 chocolate-almond clusters

Coffee or tea

MONDAY

●

BREAKFAST

Coffee, tea, tomato juice, or milk

Cottage cheese and chopped peach

1 slice of Green Banana–Nut Bread (see page 159)

LUNCH

Milk or water

SALAD: spinach, bacon bits, Parmesan cheese, and walnuts with dressing: vinegar and olive oil

1 slice of bread dipped in olive oil

Coffee or tea

SNACK

Almonds

DINNER

Red wine, milk, or water

SALAD: iceberg lettuce, tomato, and assorted vegetables with blue cheese dressing and sprinkled with vinegar

Pork chops

½ cup navy beans

Broccoli

DESSERT: Strawberries with Bittersweet-Chocolate Sauce (see page 203)

Coffee or tea

TUESDAY

●

BREAKFAST

Coffee, tea, tomato juice, or milk

½ grapefruit

Broccoli and Cheese Mini Frittatas (see page 154)

LUNCH

Diet soda or milk

Almonds

Turkey, ham, and avocado with low-carb tortilla wrap

Coffee or tea

DINNER

APPETIZER: Cheese

White wine, milk, or water

Cucumber and Vinegar Salad (see page 181)

Asparagus with butter and lemon juice

Mediterranean Baked Cod (see page 197)

½ cup rice

DESSERT: unsweetened yogurt and berries sweetened
with ½ teaspoon sugar

Coffee or tea

WEDNESDAY

●

BREAKFAST

Tomato juice or milk

Omelet with cheese, leftover asparagus, bacon bits,
and tomato

1 slice of toast with butter and 1 teaspoon jam

Coffee or tea

LUNCH

White wine, milk, or water

Chicken Caesar salad

Dark chocolate

Coffee or tea

DINNER

APPETIZER: mixed nuts

Red wine, beer, milk, or water

Taco salad

6 tortilla chips

DESSERT: $\frac{1}{4}$ cup premium ice cream sprinkled with
2 tablespoons chia seeds

Coffee or tea

THURSDAY

●

BREAKFAST

Coffee, tea, tomato juice, or milk

2 scrambled eggs, microwaved and topped with butter, salt, and pepper

1 slice Green Banana–Nut Bread (see page 159)

LUNCH

Diet soda, milk, or water

Hot dog with low-carb tortilla as bun

Apple slices

Coffee or tea

SNACK

Cheese

DINNER

APPETIZER: Spicy Bean Salad (see page 182)

White wine, milk, or water

Crispy Prosciutto-Crusted Chicken (see page 195)

Broccoli

Fauxtatoes (see page 201)

Butter

DESSERT: Carrot Cake Cupcake (see page 208)

Coffee or tea

FRIDAY

●

BREAKFAST

Coffee, tea, tomato juice, or milk

Orange slices

Breakfast Pizza (see page 155)

LUNCH

Diet soda, milk, or water

Smoked Turkey, Apple, and Grape Salad (see page 163)

1 slice of bread with butter

Coffee or tea

SNACK

Almonds

DINNER

White wine, water, or milk

SALAD: spinach, bacon bits, walnuts, mushrooms,
egg crumbles, and goat cheese with dressing:
vinegar and olive oil

Brussels sprouts

Grilled swordfish

½ boiled new potato with butter

DESSERT: dark chocolate

Coffee or tea

SATURDAY

●

BREAKFAST

Coffee, tea, or milk

½ grapefruit

Salmon Bruschetta (see page 156)

LUNCH

Diet soda, milk, or water

1 Shrimp Salad Wrap (see page 171)

Coffee or tea

SNACK

Cheese

DINNER

White wine, beer, or milk

APPETIZER: Warm Red Cabbage Salad (see page 183)

Cauliflower

Fried chicken

½ cup mashed potatoes with butter and
2 tablespoons chia seeds

DESSERT: apple slices sprinkled with cinnamon

Coffee or tea

SUNDAY

●

BREAKFAST

Coffee, tea, or milk

Berries sprinkled with $\frac{1}{2}$ teaspoon sugar, mixed with unsweetened yogurt

2 slices bacon

Omelet with cheese, tomato, and vegetable leftovers

LUNCH

Water, diet soda, or milk

Ham and Swiss Salad (see page 164)

1 slice of bread

Coffee or tea

SNACK

Cucumber and Vinegar Salad (see page 181)

DINNER

APPETIZER: peanuts

Red wine, beer, milk, or water

Steamed artichoke

Buffalo Chili (see page 191)

6 tortilla chips

DESSERT: $\frac{1}{4}$ cup premium ice cream sprinkled with 2 tablespoons chia seeds

Coffee or tea

APPENDIX

B

SUGAR BLOCKERS
DIET JOURNAL

I N CHAPTER 8, you learned a number of different ways you can tell if sugar blocking is working for you. A glucometer can be a handy tool for determining if, and how much, your blood sugar levels are spiking after meals. To see how much weight you've lost, all you need is a scale. And to see how these changes affect your energy, mood, and over-all health, you may want to track your progress as you start sugar block-ing. All of our test panelists did this, and many found it a motivating and eye-opening experience to have a written record of their success.

On the following pages, you will find 2 weeks' worth of journal pages, along with room to record your starting measurements. Each day there is space for you to record your meals and exercise activities. This may seem tedious at first, but several successful test panelists said that writ-ing down their meals and workouts helped them both be accountable and reach their goals. Also, making note of how you feel before and after you eat starch-filled meals, with or without sugar blockers, can help you identify which sugar blockers are most effective for you. You may also want to keep tabs on the glycemic load of your favorite foods. It's cer-tainly not necessary to total the GL of every meal. But if you're curious, use the list in Appendix C to help you find the estimated value of differ-ent foods. Remember: A good rule of thumb is to stay under 500 per day.

You'll see that there's also space provided to record your blood sugar levels if you choose. If you are concerned about your glucose levels and your risk of prediabetes or diabetes, measuring these levels can help you experiment and understand your blood sugar spikes. You will be able to determine which foods cause your blood sugar to spike and which ones keep it at a manageable level.

HOW TO USE A **Glucometer**

YOU DON'T have to have diabetes to gain useful information by measuring your blood sugar. Glucometers, which can be picked up at any pharmacy, come with easy-to-follow instructions. If you don't have diabetes, a good way to tell how much your blood sugar should rise after meals is to check it a few times after you eat something starchy— say, a few slices of bread or a serving of french fries—and then try to keep your after-meal readings below that level. A reasonable goal is to keep your blood sugar from rising more than 40 points from where it was before you ate. If you have diabetes, you should aim to keep your after-meal levels below 160. Levels of 160 to 200 are okay but not ideal; more than 200 is unhealthy.

When you reduce the glycemic load of the carbohydrates you eat and start using sugar blockers, you may notice a paradox: Sometimes your blood sugar after you eat will be lower than it is the next morning. The reason is that instead of rushing into your bloodstream all at once, glucose is still trickling into your bloodstream several hours later. That's a sign that you are, indeed, slowing the absorption of glucose into your bloodstream.

READY, SET, BLOCK!

TO BEGIN, enter your health measures in the spaces provided. Knowing your starting numbers will give you something to measure your progress against—and you will be seeing progress in no time.

TODAY'S DATE:

HEIGHT:

WEIGHT:

BODY MASS INDEX (BMI)*:

For the inch measurements below, you may want a friend or your spouse to help you get the most accurate numbers. While measuring, be sure to stand up straight with your shoulders back and arms relaxed. Follow these guidelines for where to measure.

CHEST: the fullest point of your bust.

WAIST: the narrowest part of your torso (usually about 2 inches above your belly button).

HIPS: the fullest part, and make sure the tape measure is parallel to the ground all the way around your hips.

ARMS AND THIGHS: the fullest part of each, with your limbs relaxed, arms hanging down, and feet shoulder-width apart.

CHEST:

WAIST:

HIPS:

LEFT BICEPS: RIGHT BICEPS:

LEFT THIGH: RIGHT THIGH:

For the following measurements, you will need to see your doctor. Since it's a good idea to check in with a physician before you start any diet or fitness program anyway, now is a good time for a checkup! You may also want to make an appointment for a few weeks down the road so that the two of you can review your sugar-blocking success.

BLOOD PRESSURE:

FASTING BLOOD GLUCOSE AND/OR A1C LEVEL:

LDL CHOLESTEROL:

HDL CHOLESTEROL:

TOTAL CHOLESTEROL:

TRIGLYCERIDE:

*To calculate your BMI, multiply your weight in pounds by 703. Divide that number by your height in inches. Divide that number by your height in inches again. Or use the BMI calculator on Prevention's Web site: www.prevention.com/bmi.

FOOD LOG

WEEK: DAY: TODAY'S DATE:

MEAL/TIME	FOOD/DRINK	ESTIMATED GLYCEMIC LOAD (OPTIONAL)	STARCH (IF ANY)	SUGAR-BLOCKING STRATEGY (IF ANY)
BREAKFAST				
SNACK				
LUNCH				
SNACK				
DINNER				

GLUCOMETER READINGS (OPTIONAL)

TIME OF DAY	LEVEL	NOTES

▶ **HOW'S YOUR MOOD?** (1 = grouchy; 10 = smiling for no apparent reason)

1   2   3   4   5   6   7   8   9   10

EXERCISE LOG

CARDIO EXERCISE	NO. OF MINUTES	STRENGTH TRAINING	NO. OF REPS	WEIGHT USED

NOTES AND OBSERVATIONS:

_____

_____

_____

_____

_____

_____

_____

▶ **HOW'S YOUR ENERGY LEVEL?** (1 = slow and sluggish; 10 = ready to take on the day!)

1   2   3   4   5   6   7   8   9   10

FOOD LOG

WEEK: DAY: _____   TODAY'S DATE: _____

MEAL/TIME	FOOD/DRINK	ESTIMATED GLYCEMIC LOAD (OPTIONAL)	STARCH (IF ANY)	SUGAR-BLOCKING STRATEGY (IF ANY)
BREAKFAST				
SNACK				
LUNCH				
SNACK				
DINNER				

GLUCOMETER READINGS (OPTIONAL)

TIME OF DAY	LEVEL	NOTES

▶ **HOW'S YOUR MOOD?** (1 = grouchy; 10 = smiling for no apparent reason)

1   2   3   4   5   6   7   8   9   10

EXERCISE LOG

CARDIO EXERCISE	NO. OF MINUTES	STRENGTH TRAINING	NO. OF REPS	WEIGHT USED

NOTES AND OBSERVATIONS:

_____

_____

_____

_____

_____

_____

_____

▶ **HOW'S YOUR ENERGY LEVEL?** (1 = slow and sluggish; 10 = ready to take on the day!)

1   2   3   4   5   6   7   8   9   10

FOOD LOG

WEEK: DAY:

MEAL/TIME	FOOD/DRINK	ESTIMATED GLYCEMIC LOAD (OPTIONAL)	STARCH (IF ANY)	SUGAR-BLOCKING STRATEGY (IF ANY)
BREAKFAST				
SNACK				
LUNCH				
SNACK				
DINNER				

GLUCOMETER READINGS (OPTIONAL)

TIME OF DAY	LEVEL	NOTES

▶ **HOW'S YOUR MOOD?** (1 = grouchy; 10 = smiling for no apparent reason)

1   2   3   4   5   6   7   8   9   10

EXERCISE LOG

CARDIO EXERCISE	NO. OF MINUTES	STRENGTH TRAINING	NO. OF REPS	WEIGHT USED

NOTES AND OBSERVATIONS:

_____

_____

_____

_____

_____

_____

_____

▶ **HOW'S YOUR ENERGY LEVEL?** (1 = slow and sluggish; 10 = ready to take on the day!)

1   2   3   4   5   6   7   8   9   10

FOOD LOG

WEEK: DAY: _____

MEAL/TIME	FOOD/DRINK	ESTIMATED GLYCEMIC LOAD (OPTIONAL)	STARCH (IF ANY)	SUGAR-BLOCKING STRATEGY (IF ANY)
BREAKFAST				
SNACK				
LUNCH				
SNACK				
DINNER				

GLUCOMETER READINGS (OPTIONAL)

TIME OF DAY	LEVEL	NOTES

▶ **HOW'S YOUR MOOD?** (1 = grouchy; 10 = smiling for no apparent reason)

1   2   3   4   5   6   7   8   9   10

EXERCISE LOG

CARDIO EXERCISE	NO. OF MINUTES	STRENGTH TRAINING	NO. OF REPS	WEIGHT USED

NOTES AND OBSERVATIONS:

▶ **HOW'S YOUR ENERGY LEVEL?** (1 = slow and sluggish; 10 = ready to take on the day!)

1   2   3   4   5   6   7   8   9   10

FOOD LOG

WEEK: DAY:

MEAL/TIME	FOOD/DRINK	ESTIMATED GLYCEMIC LOAD (OPTIONAL)	STARCH (IF ANY)	SUGAR-BLOCKING STRATEGY (IF ANY)
BREAKFAST				
SNACK				
LUNCH				
SNACK				
DINNER				

GLUCOMETER READINGS (OPTIONAL)

TIME OF DAY	LEVEL	NOTES

▶ **HOW'S YOUR MOOD?** (1 = grouchy; 10 = smiling for no apparent reason)

1   2   3   4   5   6   7   8   9   10

EXERCISE LOG

CARDIO EXERCISE	NO. OF MINUTES	STRENGTH TRAINING	NO. OF REPS	WEIGHT USED

NOTES AND OBSERVATIONS:

_____

_____

_____

_____

_____

_____

_____

▶ **HOW'S YOUR ENERGY LEVEL?** (1 = slow and sluggish; 10 = ready to take on the day!)

1   2   3   4   5   6   7   8   9   10

FOOD LOG

WEEK: DAY: TODAY'S DATE:

MEAL/TIME	FOOD/DRINK	ESTIMATED GLYCEMIC LOAD (OPTIONAL)	STARCH (IF ANY)	SUGAR-BLOCKING STRATEGY (IF ANY)
BREAKFAST				
SNACK				
LUNCH				
SNACK				
DINNER				

GLUCOMETER READINGS (OPTIONAL)

TIME OF DAY	LEVEL	NOTES

▶ **HOW'S YOUR MOOD?** (1 = grouchy; 10 = smiling for no apparent reason)

1   2   3   4   5   6   7   8   9   10

EXERCISE LOG

CARDIO EXERCISE	NO. OF MINUTES	STRENGTH TRAINING	NO. OF REPS	WEIGHT USED

NOTES AND OBSERVATIONS:

▶ **HOW'S YOUR ENERGY LEVEL?** (1 = slow and sluggish; 10 = ready to take on the day!)

1   2   3   4   5   6   7   8   9   10

FOOD LOG

WEEK: DAY: TODAY'S DATE:

MEAL/TIME	FOOD/DRINK	ESTIMATED GLYCEMIC LOAD (OPTIONAL)	STARCH (IF ANY)	SUGAR-BLOCKING STRATEGY (IF ANY)
BREAKFAST				
SNACK				
LUNCH				
SNACK				
DINNER				

GLUCOMETER READINGS (OPTIONAL)

TIME OF DAY	LEVEL	NOTES

▶ **HOW'S YOUR MOOD?** (1 = grouchy; 10 = smiling for no apparent reason)

1   2   3   4   5   6   7   8   9   10

EXERCISE LOG

CARDIO EXERCISE	NO. OF MINUTES	STRENGTH TRAINING	NO. OF REPS	WEIGHT USED

NOTES AND OBSERVATIONS:

_____

_____

_____

_____

_____

_____

_____

▶ **HOW'S YOUR ENERGY LEVEL?** (1 = slow and sluggish; 10 = ready to take on the day!)

1   2   3   4   5   6   7   8   9   10

WEEKLY MEASUREMENT RECAP

WEIGHT: _____

LEFT THIGH: _____

CHEST: _____

RIGHT THIGH: _____

WAIST: _____

LEFT BICEPS: _____

HIPS: _____

RIGHT BICEPS: _____

WEEKLY REFLECTION

USE THIS SPACE to write down any thoughts or feelings about your sugar-blocking success thus far. How have you been feeling? Have you noticed any correlation between what you're eating and your mood, attention span, stress or energy levels, or overall health? Have you hit any challenges or reached new goals?

_____

_____

_____

_____

_____

_____

_____

_____

_____

_____

FOOD LOG

WEEK: DAY: _____   TODAY'S DATE: _____

MEAL/TIME	FOOD/DRINK	ESTIMATED GLYCEMIC LOAD (OPTIONAL)	STARCH (IF ANY)	SUGAR-BLOCKING STRATEGY (IF ANY)
BREAKFAST				
SNACK				
LUNCH				
SNACK				
DINNER				

GLUCOMETER READINGS (OPTIONAL)

TIME OF DAY	LEVEL	NOTES

▶ **HOW'S YOUR MOOD?** (1 = grouchy; 10 = smiling for no apparent reason)

1   2   3   4   5   6   7   8   9   10

EXERCISE LOG

CARDIO EXERCISE	NO. OF MINUTES	STRENGTH TRAINING	NO. OF REPS	WEIGHT USED

NOTES AND OBSERVATIONS:

_____

_____

_____

_____

_____

_____

_____

▶ **HOW'S YOUR ENERGY LEVEL?** (1 = slow and sluggish; 10 = ready to take on the day!)

1   2   3   4   5   6   7   8   9   10

FOOD LOG

WEEK: DAY: TODAY'S DATE:

MEAL/TIME	FOOD/DRINK	ESTIMATED GLYCEMIC LOAD (OPTIONAL)	STARCH (IF ANY)	SUGAR-BLOCKING STRATEGY (IF ANY)
BREAKFAST				
SNACK				
LUNCH				
SNACK				
DINNER				

GLUCOMETER READINGS (OPTIONAL)

TIME OF DAY	LEVEL	NOTES

▶ **HOW'S YOUR MOOD?** (1 = grouchy; 10 = smiling for no apparent reason)

1   2   3   4   5   6   7   8   9   10

EXERCISE LOG

CARDIO EXERCISE	NO. OF MINUTES	STRENGTH TRAINING	NO. OF REPS	WEIGHT USED

NOTES AND OBSERVATIONS:

_____

_____

_____

_____

_____

_____

▶ **HOW'S YOUR ENERGY LEVEL?** (1 = slow and sluggish; 10 = ready to take on the day!)

1   2   3   4   5   6   7   8   9   10

FOOD LOG

WEEK: DAY:

TODAY'S DATE:

MEAL/TIME	FOOD/DRINK	ESTIMATED GLYCEMIC LOAD (OPTIONAL)	STARCH (IF ANY)	SUGAR-BLOCKING STRATEGY (IF ANY)
BREAKFAST				
SNACK				
LUNCH				
SNACK				
DINNER				

GLUCOMETER READINGS (OPTIONAL)

TIME OF DAY	LEVEL	NOTES

▶ **HOW'S YOUR MOOD?** (1 = grouchy; 10 = smiling for no apparent reason)

1   2   3   4   5   6   7   8   9   10

EXERCISE LOG

CARDIO EXERCISE	NO. OF MINUTES	STRENGTH TRAINING	NO. OF REPS	WEIGHT USED

NOTES AND OBSERVATIONS:

▶ **HOW'S YOUR ENERGY LEVEL?** (1 = slow and sluggish; 10 = ready to take on the day!)

1   2   3   4   5   6   7   8   9   10

FOOD LOG

WEEK: DAY: 　 TODAY'S DATE:

MEAL/TIME	FOOD/DRINK	ESTIMATED GLYCEMIC LOAD (OPTIONAL)	STARCH (IF ANY)	SUGAR-BLOCKING STRATEGY (IF ANY)
BREAKFAST				
SNACK				
LUNCH				
SNACK				
DINNER				

GLUCOMETER READINGS (OPTIONAL)

TIME OF DAY	LEVEL	NOTES

▶ **HOW'S YOUR MOOD?** (1 = grouchy; 10 = smiling for no apparent reason)

1　　2　　3　　4　　5　　6　　7　　8　　9　　10

EXERCISE LOG

CARDIO EXERCISE	NO. OF MINUTES	STRENGTH TRAINING	NO. OF REPS	WEIGHT USED

NOTES AND OBSERVATIONS:

_____

_____

_____

_____

_____

_____

_____

▶ **HOW'S YOUR ENERGY LEVEL?** (1 = slow and sluggish; 10 = ready to take on the day!)

1   2   3   4   5   6   7   8   9   10

FOOD LOG

WEEK: DAY:

TODAY'S DATE:

MEAL/TIME	FOOD/DRINK	ESTIMATED GLYCEMIC LOAD (OPTIONAL)	STARCH (IF ANY)	SUGAR-BLOCKING STRATEGY (IF ANY)
BREAKFAST				
SNACK				
LUNCH				
SNACK				
DINNER				

GLUCOMETER READINGS (OPTIONAL)

TIME OF DAY	LEVEL	NOTES

▶ **HOW'S YOUR MOOD?** (1 = grouchy; 10 = smiling for no apparent reason)

   1   2   3   4   5   6   7   8   9   10

EXERCISE LOG

CARDIO EXERCISE	NO. OF MINUTES	STRENGTH TRAINING	NO. OF REPS	WEIGHT USED

NOTES AND OBSERVATIONS:

▶ **HOW'S YOUR ENERGY LEVEL?** (1 = slow and sluggish; 10 = ready to take on the day!)

1   2   3   4   5   6   7   8   9   10

FOOD LOG

WEEK: DAY: _____

MEAL/TIME	FOOD/DRINK	ESTIMATED GLYCEMIC LOAD (OPTIONAL)	STARCH (IF ANY)	SUGAR-BLOCKING STRATEGY (IF ANY)
BREAKFAST				
SNACK				
LUNCH				
SNACK				
DINNER				

GLUCOMETER READINGS (OPTIONAL)

TIME OF DAY	LEVEL	NOTES

▶ **HOW'S YOUR MOOD?** (1 = grouchy; 10 = smiling for no apparent reason)

1   2   3   4   5   6   7   8   9   10

EXERCISE LOG

CARDIO EXERCISE	NO. OF MINUTES	STRENGTH TRAINING	NO. OF REPS	WEIGHT USED

NOTES AND OBSERVATIONS:

_____

_____

_____

_____

_____

_____

_____

▶ **HOW'S YOUR ENERGY LEVEL?** (1 = slow and sluggish; 10 = ready to take on the day!)

1   2   3   4   5   6   7   8   9   10

FOOD LOG

WEEK:　　DAY: TODAY'S DATE:

MEAL/TIME	FOOD/DRINK	ESTIMATED GLYCEMIC LOAD (OPTIONAL)	STARCH (IF ANY)	SUGAR-BLOCKING STRATEGY (IF ANY)
BREAKFAST				
SNACK				
LUNCH				
SNACK				
DINNER				

GLUCOMETER READINGS (OPTIONAL)

TIME OF DAY	LEVEL	NOTES

▶ **HOW'S YOUR MOOD?** (1 = grouchy; 10 = smiling for no apparent reason)

1　　2　　3　　4　　5　　6　　7　　8　　9　　10

EXERCISE LOG

CARDIO EXERCISE	NO. OF MINUTES	STRENGTH TRAINING	NO. OF REPS	WEIGHT USED

NOTES AND OBSERVATIONS:

▶ **HOW'S YOUR ENERGY LEVEL?** (1 = slow and sluggish; 10 = ready to take on the day!)

1   2   3   4   5   6   7   8   9   10

WEEKLY MEASUREMENT RECAP

WEIGHT: _____

LEFT THIGH: _____

CHEST: _____

RIGHT THIGH: _____

WAIST: _____

LEFT BICEPS: _____

HIPS: _____

RIGHT BICEPS: _____

WEEKLY REFLECTION

USE THIS SPACE to write down any thoughts or feelings about your sugar-blocking success thus far. How have you been feeling? Have you noticed any correlation between what you're eating and your mood, attention span, stress or energy levels, or overall health? Have you hit any challenges or reached new goals?

_____

_____

_____

_____

_____

_____

_____

_____

_____

_____

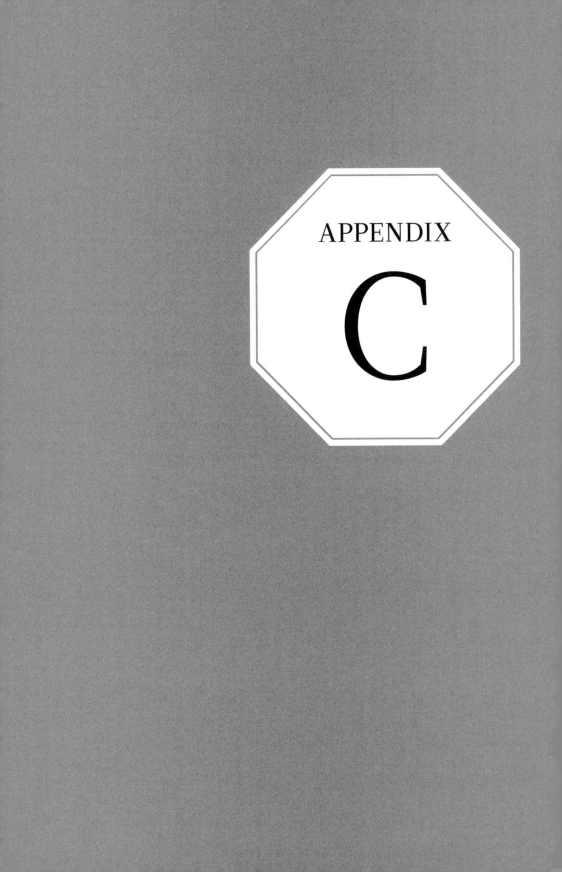

APPENDIX

C

LIST OF GLYCEMIC LOADS

(expressed as the percentage of that of a slice of white bread)

FOOD ITEM	DESCRIPTION	AVAILABLE CARBOHYDRATE (PERCENT)	TYPICAL AMERICAN SERVING	GLYCEMIC LOAD
Baked Goods				
Oatmeal cookie	1 medium	68	1 oz	102
Apple muffin, sugarless	2½" diameter	32	2½ oz	107
Cookie, average, all types	1 medium	64	1 oz	114
Croissant	1 medium	46	1½ oz	127
Crumpet	1 medium	38	2 oz	148
Bran muffin	2½" diameter	42	2 oz	149
Pastry	Average serving	46	2 oz	149
Chocolate cake	1 slice (4" × 4" × 1")	47	3 oz	154
Vanilla wafers	4 wafers	72	1 oz	159
Graham cracker	1 rectangle	72	1 oz	159
Blueberry muffin	2½" diameter	51	2 oz	169
Carrot cake	1 square (3" × 3" × 1½")	56	2 oz	199
Carrot muffin	2½" diameter	56	2 oz	199
Waffle	7" diameter	37	2½ oz	203
Doughnut	1 medium	49	2 oz	205
Cupcake	2½" diameter	68	1½ oz	213
Angel food cake	1 slice (4" × 4" × 1")	58	2 oz	216
English muffin	1 medium	47	2 oz	224
Pound cake	1 slice (4" × 4" × 1")	53	3 oz	241

(continued)

FOOD ITEM	DESCRIPTION	AVAILABLE CARBOHYDRATE (PERCENT)	TYPICAL AMERICAN SERVING	GLYCEMIC LOAD
Baked Goods (continued)				
Corn muffin	2½" diameter	51	2 oz	299
Pancake	5" diameter	73	2½ oz	346
Alcoholic Beverages				
Spirits	1½ oz	0	1½ oz	<15
Red wine	6-oz glass	0	6 oz	<15
White wine	6-oz glass	0	6 oz	<15
Beer	12-oz can/bottle	3	12 oz	70
Nonalcoholic Beverages				
Tomato juice	6-oz glass	4	6 oz	27
V8 juice	6-oz glass	4	6 oz	27
Carrot juice	6-oz glass	12	6 oz	68
Grapefruit juice, unsweetened	6-oz glass	9	6 oz	75
Apple juice, unsweetened	6-oz glass	12	6 oz	82
Chocolate milk	8-oz glass	10	8 oz	82
Orange juice	6-oz glass	10	6 oz	89
Prune juice	6-oz glass	14	6 oz	102
Cranberry juice	6-oz glass	12	6 oz	109
Pineapple juice, unsweetened	6-oz glass	14	6 oz	109
Raspberry smoothie	8-oz glass	16	8 oz	127
Lemonade	8-oz glass	11	8 oz	136
Ensure	8-oz glass	17	8 oz	182
Coca-Cola	12-oz can	10	12 oz	218
Gatorade	20-oz bottle	6	20 oz	273
Orange soda	12-oz glass	14	12 oz	314

FOOD ITEM	DESCRIPTION	AVAILABLE CARBOHYDRATE (PERCENT)	TYPICAL AMERICAN SERVING	GLYCEMIC LOAD
Breads and Rolls				
Tortilla (wheat)	1 medium	52	$1\frac{3}{8}$ oz	64
Pizza crust	1 slice	22	$3\frac{1}{2}$ oz	70
Tortilla (corn)	1 medium	48	$1\frac{1}{4}$ oz	87
White bread	$\frac{1}{2}$" slice	47	1 oz	107
Whole meal rye bread	$\frac{3}{8}$" slice	40	2 oz	114
Sourdough bread	$\frac{3}{8}$" slice	47	$1\frac{1}{2}$ oz	114
Oat bran bread	$\frac{3}{8}$" slice	60	$1\frac{1}{2}$ oz	128
Whole wheat bread	$\frac{1}{2}$" slice	43	$1\frac{1}{2}$ oz	129
Rye bread	$\frac{3}{8}$" slice	47	$1\frac{1}{2}$ oz	142
Banana bread, sugarless	1 slice (4" × 4" × 1")	48	3 oz	170
80% whole kernel oat bread	$\frac{3}{8}$" slice	63	$1\frac{1}{2}$ oz	170
Buckwheat bread	$\frac{3}{8}$" slice	63	$1\frac{1}{2}$ oz	183
80% whole kernel barley bread	$\frac{3}{8}$" slice	67	$1\frac{1}{2}$ oz	185
Pita	8" diameter	57	2 oz	189
Hamburger bun	Top and bottom, 5" diameter	50	$2\frac{1}{2}$ oz	213
80% whole kernel wheat bread	$\frac{3}{8}$" slice	67	$2\frac{1}{4}$ oz	213
French bread	$\frac{1}{2}$" slice	50	2 oz	284
Bagel	1 medium	50	$3\frac{1}{3}$ oz	340
Breakfast Cereals				
All-Bran	$\frac{1}{2}$ cup	77	1 oz	85
Muesli	1 cup	53	1 oz	95

(continued)

FOOD ITEM	DESCRIPTION	AVAILABLE CARBOHYDRATE (PERCENT)	TYPICAL AMERICAN SERVING	GLYCEMIC LOAD
Breakfast Cereals (continued)				
Oatmeal (from rolled oats)	1 cup	10	8 oz	123
Special K	1 cup	70	1 oz	133
Cheerios	1 cup	40	1 oz	142
Shredded wheat	1 cup	67	1 oz	142
Grape-Nuts	1 cup	70	1 oz	142
Granola	1 cup	87	1 oz	142
Puffed wheat	1 cup	70	1 oz	151
Kashi	1 cup	80	1 oz	151
Instant oatmeal	1 cup	10	8 oz	154
Cream of Wheat, cooked	1 cup	10	8 oz	154
Total	1 cup	73	1 oz	161
Froot Loops	1 cup	87	1 oz	170
Cornflakes	1 cup	77	1 oz	199
Rice Krispies	1 cup	87	1 oz	208
Rice Chex	1 cup	87	1 oz	218
Raisin bran	1 cup	63	2 oz	227
Candy and Snacks				
Sugar-free milk chocolate	2 squares (1" × 1" × ¼")	30	1 oz	17
Life Saver	1 piece	100	$\frac{1}{10}$ oz	20
Peanut M&M's	1 snack-size package	57	$\frac{3}{4}$ oz	43
Dark chocolate	2 squares (1" × 1" × ¼")	52	1 oz	44
Licorice	1 twist	70	$\frac{1}{3}$ oz	45

FOOD ITEM	DESCRIPTION	AVAILABLE CARBOHYDRATE (PERCENT)	TYPICAL AMERICAN SERVING	GLYCEMIC LOAD
Candy and Snacks *(continued)*				
White chocolate	2 squares (1″ × 1″ × ¼″)	44	⅔ oz	49
Milk chocolate	2 squares (1″ × 1″ × ¼″)	44	1 oz	68
Jelly beans	6 beans	93	½ oz	104
Granola bar, apple or cranberry	1 bar	77	1 oz	131
Snickers bar	1 regular-size bar	57	2 oz	218
Chips and Crackers				
Potato chips	Small bag	42	1 oz	62
Corn chips	1 package	52	1 oz	97
Popcorn	4 cups	55	1 oz	114
Rye crisp	1 rectangle	64	1 oz	125
Wheat Thins	4 small	68	1 oz	136
Soda crackers	2 regular size	68	1 oz	136
Pretzels	Small bag	67	1 oz	151
Rice cakes	3 regular size	84	1 oz	190
Dairy Products				
Cheese	2″ × 2″ × 1″ slice	0	2 oz	<15
Butter	1 Tbsp	0	¼ oz	<15
Margarine	Typical serving	0	¼ oz	<15
Sour cream	Typical serving	0	2 oz	<15
Yogurt, full-fat (unsweetened)	½ cup	5	4 oz	17
Milk (whole)	8-oz glass	5	8 oz	37

(continued)

FOOD ITEM	DESCRIPTION	AVAILABLE CARBOHYDRATE (PERCENT)	TYPICAL AMERICAN SERVING	GLYCEMIC LOAD
Dairy Products *(continued)*				
Milk (fat-free)	8-oz glass	5	8 oz	41
Yogurt, low-fat (sweetened)	½ cup	16	4 oz	57
Soy milk	8-oz glass	7	8 oz	62
Vanilla ice cream (high fat)	½ cup	18	4 oz	68
Chocolate milk (low-fat)	8-oz glass	10	8 oz	82
Custard	½ cup	17	4½ oz	89
Chocolate pudding	½ cup	16	4½ oz	89
Chocolate ice cream (high-fat)	½ cup	18	4½ oz	91
Vanilla ice cream (low fat)	½ cup	36	4 oz	159
Frozen tofu	½ cup	30	4 oz	379
Fruit				
Strawberries	1 cup	3	5½ oz	13
Apricot	1 medium	8	2 oz	24
Grapefruit	1 half	9	4½ oz	32
Plum	1 medium	10	3 oz	36
Nectarine	1 medium	8	4 oz	38
Cherries, dark	8	12	2 oz	43
Kiwifruit	1 medium	10	3 oz	43
Peaches, canned in natural juice	½ cup	10	4 oz	45
Peach, fresh	1 medium	9	4 oz	47
Grapes	½ cup	15	2½ oz	47

FOOD ITEM	DESCRIPTION	AVAILABLE CARBOHYDRATE (PERCENT)	TYPICAL AMERICAN SERVING	GLYCEMIC LOAD
Fruit *(continued)*				
Pineapple	1 slice ($^3/_4$" × $3^1/_2$" wide)	11	3 oz	50
Watermelon	1 cup cubed	5	$5^1/_2$ oz	52
Cantaloupe	1 cup cubed	5	$5^1/_2$ oz	52
Pear	1 medium	9	6 oz	57
Mango	$^1/_2$ cup	14	3 oz	57
Orange	1 medium	9	6 oz	71
Apricot, dried	2 oz	45	2 oz	76
Apple	1 medium	13	$5^1/_2$ oz	78
Banana	1 medium	17	$3^1/_4$ oz	85
Prunes, pitted, dried	2 oz	55	2 oz	95
Apple, dried	2 oz	60	2 oz	104
Peaches, canned in heavy syrup	$^1/_2$ cup	16	4 oz	112
Raisins	2 Tbsp	73	1 oz	133
Figs	3 medium	43	2 oz	151
Dates	5 medium	67	$1^1/_2$ oz	298
Meat, Poultry, and Fish				
Beef	10-oz steak	0	10 oz	<15
Pork	Two 5-oz chops	0	10 oz	<15
Chicken	1 breast	0	10 oz	<15
Fish	8-oz fillet	0	8 oz	<15
Lamb	Three 4-oz chops	0	12 oz	<15

(continued)

FOOD ITEM	DESCRIPTION	AVAILABLE CARBOHYDRATE (PERCENT)	TYPICAL AMERICAN SERVING	GLYCEMIC LOAD
Mixed Meals				
Deluxe burger, no bun	1 medium	16	3¼ oz	<15
Pizza, minus outer rim of crust	1 slice	12	3 oz	45
Wheat tortilla, bean-filled	1 burrito	18	4 oz	50
Chicken nuggets	4 oz	16	4 oz	70
Deluxe burger, minus top bun	1 medium	8	4¼ oz	80
Cannelloni, spinach, ricotta	2 tubes	18	12 oz	88
Pizza, crust intact	1 slice	24	4 oz	90
Chili con carne	1 cup	12	8 oz	91
Veggie burger	1 medium	24	3½ oz	140
Deluxe hamburger	1 medium	16	5¾ oz	170
Filet-O-Fish sandwich	1 medium	30	4½ oz	200
Chicken korma and rice	10 oz	16	10 oz	210
McChicken sandwich	1 medium	22	6½ oz	260
Nuts				
Peanuts	¼ cup	8	1¼ oz	<15
Walnuts	¼ cup	8	1¼ oz	<15
Almonds	¼ cup	8	1¼ oz	<15
Cashews	¼ cup	26	1¼ oz	21
Pasta				
Asian bean noodles	1 cup	25	5 oz	118
Spaghetti, whole grain	1 cup	23	5 oz	126

FOOD ITEM	DESCRIPTION	AVAILABLE CARBOHYDRATE (PERCENT)	TYPICAL AMERICAN SERVING	GLYCEMIC LOAD
Pasta *(continued)*				
Vermicelli	1 cup	24	5 oz	126
Spaghetti (boiled 5 min)	1 cup	27	5 oz	142
Fettuccine	1 cup	23	5 oz	142
Noodles (instant, boiled 2 min)	1 cup	22	5 oz	150
Capellini	1 cup	25	5 oz	158
Spaghetti (boiled 10–15 min)	1 cup	27	5 oz	166
Linguine	1 cup	25	5 oz	181
Macaroni	1 cup	28	5 oz	181
Rice noodles	1 cup	22	5 oz	181
Spaghetti (boiled 20 min)	1 cup	24	5 oz	213
Macaroni and cheese (boxed)	1 cup	28	5 oz	252
Gnocchi	1 cup	27	5 oz	260
Soups				
Tomato soup	1 cup	7	8 oz	55
Minestrone	1 cup	7	8 oz	64
Lentil soup	1 cup	8	8 oz	82
Split-pea soup	1 cup	11	8 oz	145
Black bean soup	1 cup	11	8 oz	154
Sweeteners				
Artificial sweeteners	1 tsp		⅙ oz	<15
Honey	1 tsp	72	⅙ oz	16

(continued)

APPENDIX C

FOOD ITEM	DESCRIPTION	AVAILABLE CARBOHYDRATE (PERCENT)	TYPICAL AMERICAN SERVING	GLYCEMIC LOAD
Sweeteners *(continued)*				
Table sugar	1 rounded tsp	100	1/6 oz	28
Syrup	1/4 cup	100	2 oz	364
Vegetables, Legumes, and Grains				
Carrot (raw)	1 medium (7 1/2")	10	3 oz	11
Lettuce	1 cup	3	2 1/2 oz	<15
Spinach	1 cup	5	2 1/2 oz	<15
Cucumber	1 cup	2	6 oz	<15
Mushrooms	1/2 cup	7	2 oz	<15
Asparagus	4 spears	6	3 oz	<15
Peppers	1/2 medium	4	2 oz	<15
Broccoli	1/2 cup	6	1 1/2 oz	<15
Chickpeas, boiled	2 Tbsp	10	1 oz	<15
Tomato	1 medium	6	5 oz	<15
Peas	1/4 cup	9	1 1/2 oz	16
Chickpeas, boiled	1/2 cup	20	3 oz	17
Carrots, boiled	2/3 cup	6	3 oz	21
Fava beans	1/2 cup	6	3 oz	32
Lentils	1/2 cup	11	3 1/2 oz	33
Butter beans	1/2 cup	13	3 oz	34
Cannellini beans	1/2 cup	14	3 oz	34
Kidney beans	1/2 cup	17	3 oz	40
Navy beans	1/2 cup	10	3 oz	40
Parsnips	1/2 cup	10	3 oz	50

FOOD ITEM	DESCRIPTION	AVAILABLE CARBOHYDRATE (PERCENT)	TYPICAL AMERICAN SERVING	GLYCEMIC LOAD
Vegetables *(continued)*				
Lima beans	½ cup	12	3 oz	57
Refried pinto beans	½ cup	17	3 oz	57
Black-eyed peas	½ cup	20	3 oz	74
Yam	½ cup	24	5 oz	123
Quinoa	1 cup	17	6½ oz	160
Potato, instant mashed	¾ cup	13	5 oz	161
Sweet potato	½ cup	19	5 oz	161
Corn on the cob	1 ear	21	5⅓ oz	171
Couscous	½ cup	23	4 oz	174
French fries	Medium serving (McDonald's)	19	5¼ oz	219
Brown and wild rice mix	1 cup	26	6½ oz	221
Brown rice	1 cup	22	6½ oz	222
Baked potato	1 medium	20	5 oz	264
Basmati rice	1 cup	25	6½ oz	271
White rice	1 cup	24	6½ oz	283
Sticky white rice	1 cup	19	6½ oz	295
Miscellaneous				
Eggs	Typical serving	0	1½ oz	<15
Salad dressing	Typical serving	10	2 oz	<15
Agave	2 tsp	100	¼ oz	<15
Cane sugar	1 level tsp	100	⅛ oz	28

ACKNOWLEDGMENTS

I OWE A DEBT OF GRATITUDE to my now-retired literary agent of many years, Elizabeth Frost-Knappman, for her unwavering support, incisive advice, and impeccable judgment. I also owe thanks to my new agent, Roger Williams, who applied his considerable talents in shepherding this book through the publishing process. I have been especially impressed with the diligence and commitment demonstrated by Andrea Au Levitt, my editor at Rodale, who put in many hours of hard work on this project.

Many thanks also to our panel of testers for their time and their feedback: Joann Cheeks, Brenda Frana, Linda Frey, Jeremy Giandomenico, Joan Giandomenico, Sandi Hausman, Valerie Hayes, Jim Hobar, Tammy Hobar, Renee Marchisotto, Nancy Mikkelson, Scott Newhard, Michelle Newhard, Bruce Reiser, Cindy Swan, and Jane Wilchak. Thanks, too, to Brian Goodman of Moore Medical and Kristen Dopf of Nipro Diagnostics for donating the glucometers used by our test panelists.

Of course, I probably wouldn't be writing books if it weren't for my office manager, Shannon Pagan, and my medical assistant, Nadine Warner, who have made it possible for me to practice medicine and have the energy to write about it.

INDEX

Underscored page references indicate boxed text and tables. **Boldface** references indicate photographs.

Chest press, 248–49, **248, 249**
Chewing, in carbohydrate digestion, 45
Chia seeds, 101–2, 101
　added to bran cereal, 217
　as sugar blocker, 309
Chicken
　Chicken Cacciatore, 193
　Crispy Prosciutto-Crusted Chicken, 195
　glycemic load of, 367
　Herb-Garlic Chicken, 194
　omega-3 fatty acids in, 114
Chickpeas
　Pasta and Chickpea Salad, 168
Chili
　Buffalo Chili, 191
　Pork Chili Verde, 192
Chinese restaurants, dining guidelines
　　for, 225–26
Chips, glycemic load of, 365
Chocolate
　Chocolate Flourless Cake, 207
　as dessert, 219, 223, 226–27
　glycemic load of, 70, 71
　　estimating, 213
　Mocha Granita, 209
　Nutty Brownies, 206
　Strawberries with Bittersweet-
　　Chocolate Sauce, 203
Cholesterol, blood
　acarbose improving, 279
　desirable levels of, with diabetes,
　　292–93
　effect of nuts on, 100, 115
　functions of, 294
　HDL, 293, 297–98
　　desirable levels of, 298
　　increasing, 35, 139, 298–302
　　insulin resistance lowering, 278
　　low, 18, 19–20, 21
　　low-carbohydrate diet increasing, 84
　　recording, 327
　high
　　causes of, 82, 294
　　health risks from, 85, 291
　imbalanced, health risks from, 24
　LDL, 293, 294
　　desirable levels of, 296
　　factors increasing, 294–95
　　high, with insulin resistance, 20
　　medications reducing, 296–97
　　recording, 327

　lowering, with
　　phytosterols, 94
　　soluble fiber, 93–94
　metformin improving, 280
　monounsaturated fatty acids and, 113
　recording, 327
　reduced, in test panelists, 27, 140, 301
　total, recording, 327
Cholesterol, dietary
　diabetes and, 83
　misconceptions about, 81–82
Cholesterol-lowering medications,
　　296–97
Cholesterol-to-HDL ratio, desirable, 298
Cinnamon, reducing blood sugar, 116
Circadian-rhythm disturbances, effect on
　　blood sugar, 268–69
Civilization, diseases of, 8–9
Coconut flour, 147
Cod
　Mediterranean Baked Cod, 197
Coffee
　Mocha Granita, 209
　reducing diabetes risk, 270
Constipation, 91, 92, 103, 104
Continuous positive airway pressure
　　(CPAP) machines, 270–71
Corn, types to eliminate, 129
Corn products, types to eliminate, 129
CPAP machines, 270–71
Crab
　Curried Crab Dip, 178
Crackers, glycemic load of, 365
Cravings
　from carbohydrate elimination, 34, 35,
　　86
　stable blood sugar reducing, 139
Cucumbers
　Cucumber and Vinegar Salad, 181
　Veggie-Hummus Pita, 169
Cupcakes
　Carrot Cake Cupcakes, 208
Curry powder
　Curried Crab Dip, 178

D

Dairy products, glycemic load of,
　　365–66
Delayed sleep-phase syndrome, reducing
　　insulin sensitivity, 269

Recipes, sugar-blocking, 147–49. *See also*
        specific recipes
Repetitions, in strength training, 241, 242
Resistance bands or tubes, 242–43
Resistance training. *See* Strength training
Restaurants. *See* Dining out guidelines
Rice
    guidelines for eating, with Asian meals,
        225–26
    substitute for, 144–45
Ricotta cheese
    Creamy Pesto Ricotta, 180
    Scrambled Eggs with Pesto and
        Ricotta, 152
Rolls, glycemic load of, <u>363</u>
Rosiglitazone, <u>284</u>
Running
    benefits of, 241
    vs. walking, <u>236</u>, 237–39

S

Salad dressings. *See* Vinaigrettes
Salads
    Beef and Mushroom Stew with Carrot
        and Turnip Salad, 190
    Classic Cobb Salad, 165
    Cucumber and Vinegar Salad, 181
    with dinner, 218, 222
    with hamburger, 222
    with Italian meals, 224
    for lunch, 218
    Pasta and Chickpea Salad, 168
    sandwich fillings on, 145
    Sesame-Ginger Green Bean Salad, 184
    Shrimp Salad Wraps, 171
    Smoked Turkey, Apple, and Grape
        Salad, 163
    Somewhat Potato-and-Egg Salad, 167
    Spicy Bean Salad, 182
    Spinach and Egg Salad, 166
    with starches, 309
    as sugar blocker, 46, 51, 95, 131, 148
    Warm Red Cabbage Salad, 183
    Zucchini Salad, 185
Salmon
    Salmon Bruschetta, 156
Salt. *See also* Sodium
    high blood pressure and, 79, 80, 118–19,
        <u>304</u>
    presumed health risks from, 79, 80

Sandwiches. *See also* Wraps
    Roast Beef and Mango Roll-Ups, 170
    for typical American lunch, 217
Sauce
    Strawberries with Bittersweet-
        Chocolate Sauce, 203
Sausage
    Sausage and Peppers, 196
    Sausage Pizzas, 172
Saxagliptin, 284
Scones
    Savory Oat Scones, 177
Seated row, 256–57, **256**, **257**
Second-meal effect, from soluble fiber,
        93, 95, 97, 99
Sedentary lifestyle, insulin resistance
        from, 16–17
Seeds
    fiber content and glycemic load of, <u>101</u>,
        <u>135</u>
    starch in, <u>5</u>, 6
    sugar-blocking
        chia seeds, 101–2
        flaxseeds, 102
Sesame dressing
    Sesame-Ginger Green Bean Salad, 184
Sets, in strength training, 242
Shellfish
    Curried Crab Dip, 178
    Shrimp Salad Wraps, 171
Shirataki noodles, as pasta substitute, 144
Shortcakes
    Mixed-Berry Shortcakes, 204
Shoulder shrug, 250–51, **250**, **251**
Shrimp
    Shrimp Salad Wraps, 171
Sitagliptin, 284
Situps, 243, 244–45, **244**, **245**
Sleep
    body clock and, 268–69
    poor, reducing insulin sensitivity,
        267–68, 271
Sleep apnea, 269–71
Slow-twitch muscle fibers, 229, 232–33,
        235, 239, 241, 285
Smoking
    atherosclerosis from, 291
    health risks from, 24
Smoking cessation
    with diabetes, 292, 293
    for increasing HDL cholesterol, 301

Success stories
  Frey, Linda, 140–41, **140**, **141**
  Giandomenico, Jeremy, 300–301, **300**
  Giandomenico, Joan, 106–7, **106**, **107**
  Hausman, Sandi, 54–55, **54**, **55**
  Hayes, Valerie, 26–27, **26**, **27**
  Hobar, Jim and Tammy, 78–79, **79**
  Marchisotto, Renee, 286–87, **286**, **287**
  Newhard, Michelle, 220–21, **220**
  Swan, Cindy, 272–273, **272**, **273**
  Wilchak, Jane, 146, **146**
Sucrose, 8, 74
Sugar
  as addictive, 73
  combined with starch, 70–71
  composition of, 74
  glycemic load of, 73
  vs. high-fructose corn syrup, 72
  starch pile as, 214
  as sucrose, 8
Sugar blockers. *See also* Sugar-blocking
    systems, methods of activating
  after-meal walk, 51, 52, 121, 131, 132, 214,
    236
  alcohol, 49, 52, 119–20, 131, 132, 224,
    309
  with breakfast cereal, 217
  cell membranes as, 290
  concluding summary about, 306–7
  for diabetics, 111–12
  fat, 47, 49, 112–14, 130–31, 148
  fiber, 5, 48, 52, 95, 131, 132, 133–35
  in full-service restaurant meals, 222
  hamburger trimmings, 219
  health benefits from, 4, 43, 45, 214
  identifying most effective, 325
  in Italian restaurants, 224, 225
  in lunch salad, 218
  medications as, 276–85
  in menus, 309
  natural, 44, 57, 68
  nuts, 52, 54, 115, 139, 140
  pickles, 118–19
  power of combining, 52–53, 122–23,
    212
  for preventing sleep problems, 271
  salads, 46, 51, 95, 131, 148
  unpredictability of, 122–23
  vinegar, 52, 55, 117–18, 131, 132, 218, 224,
    309
  when to eat, 136

Sugar Blockers Diet
  basics of, 212
  gauging effectiveness of, 135–39, 325
  steps in
    avoiding culprit foods, 129–30
    identifying culprit foods, 128–29
    using sugar blockers when starches
      are unavoidable, 130–32
Sugar Blockers Diet Journal, 325–26,
    327–59
Sugar Blockers Menus, 309–23
Sugar-blocking recipes, 147–49. *See also*
    specific recipes
Sugar-blocking systems, methods of
    activating
  consuming vinegar, 117–19
  drinking alcohol, 119–20
  eating fat before meal, 112–16
  eating protein with carbs, 120
  using cinnamon, 116
  using nonstarch flours, 115–16
Sugar shocks
  from beans, 99
  from breakfast, 215
  health benefits of eliminating, 25, 305
  identifying sources of, 57
  preventing, 53, 212, 214
Sugar substitutes, 74
Sugar-sweetened beverages, 75–76
  eliminating, 87, 128, 129, 212, 309
Sushi, 226
Swan, Cindy, 102, 128, 272–273, **272**, **273**
Sweeteners
  glycemic load of, 369–70
  types of, 74
Sweets. *See also* Desserts; Snacks/
    desserts
  with low glycemic load, 73
  rules for eating, 74
  without starch, glycemic load of, 70,
    71
Symlin, 283–84

T

Tacos
  Fish Tacos, 198
Thiazolidinediones, 284
Tilapia
  Fish Tacos, 198
Toast, for breakfast, 216